Praise for *A Different Track*

"Alexandra Kitty shows us with skill and empathy what the patients, nurses and doctors thought of the hospital trains they served on and the danger and camaraderie that they experienced as the trains wove through battlefields, under strafing by enemy planes. This is an exceptionally well-referenced book and an intriguing read."

MARION McKINNON CROOK
award-winning author of *Always Pack a Candle: A Nurse in the Cariboo-Chilcotin*

"Nothing encapsulates the horror of war better than a hospital train standing in a siding near a battlefield waiting for the inevitable casualties of the conflict. *A Different Track* highlights this largely forgotten feature of warfare and shows how this service, often provided by women whose role, too, has been lost in the midst of time, saved the lives of thousands of wounded men."

CHRISTIAN WOLMAR
author of *Engines of War* and *The Liberation Line*

"Fascinating and well researched. Alexandra Kitty presents history that must be preserved."

PATRICIA W. SEWELL (COLLIER)
editor of *Healers in World War II: Oral Histories of Medical Corps Personnel*

"A fascinating look at hospital trains and the people, especially nurses, who made them work."

TERRY COPP
author of *Fields of Fire: The Canadians in Normandy*

"*A Different Track* is a love letter to the hospital trains that wound their way across Europe and North America during the Second World War. Alexandra Kitty draws on newspaper reporting of the time to trace the ways the trains offered a narrative of hope, order, and safety that was sorely needed in the dark days of the conflict."

AMY SHAW
co-editor of *Making the Best of It: Women and Girls of Canada and Newfoundland during the Second World War*

"The romance of trains collides with the bloodletting of war in a high-stakes game on rails, as told in the pages of this remarkable book. Historian Alexandra Kitty has written a scholarly yet accessible work inspired by her own grandmother's role as a nurse on a hospital train despite personal tragedy. Millions of soldiers and civilians were saved on these locomotives, despite severely limited resources—thanks to the shockingly down-and-dirty methods medical professionals had to resort to in the face of the terrors of world-wide conflict. Absorbing reading, a riveting and well-documented triumph."

JACQUELINE L. CARMICHAEL
author of *Heard Amid the Guns: True Stories from the Western Front, 1914–1918*

A DIFFERENT
TRACK

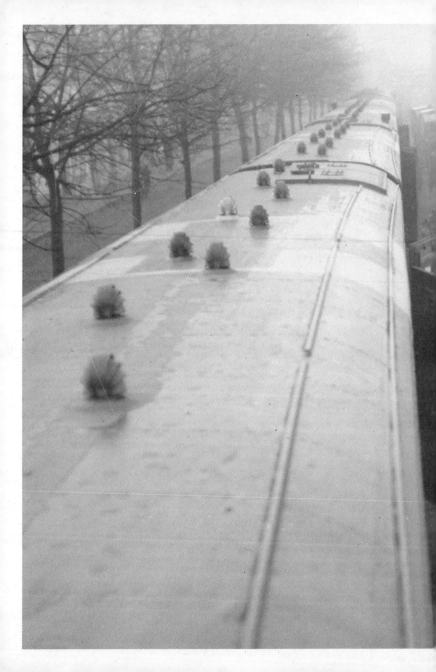

A DIFFERENT TRACK

Hospital Trains of the Second World War

Alexandra Kitty

Heritage House Publishing Company Ltd.
heritagehouse.ca

Cataloguing information available from Library and Archives Canada

978-1-77203-457-8 (paperback)
978-1-77203-458-5 (e-book)

Edited by Renée Layberry
Cover design by Setareh Ashrafologhalai
Interior design by Jacqui Thomas
Cover image: Hospital Train (1942), by Evelyn Mary Dunbar. © IWM Art.IWM ART LD 2477
Frontispiece: Wounded soldiers being loaded into a hospital train in Belgium, March 1945. IWM B 15253

The interior of this book was produced on 100% post-consumer recycled paper, processed chlorine free, and printed with vegetable-based inks.

Heritage House gratefully acknowledges that the land on which we live and work is within the traditional territories of the Lkwungen (Esquimalt and Songhees), Malahat, Pacheedaht, Scia'new, T'Sou-ke, and W̱SÁNEĆ (Pauquachin, Tsartlip, Tsawout, Tseycum) Peoples.

We acknowledge the financial support of the Government of Canada through the Canada Book Fund (CBF) and the Canada Council for the Arts, and the Province of British Columbia through the British Columbia Arts Council and the Book Publishing Tax Credit.

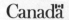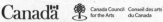

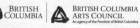

27 26 25 24 23 1 2 3 4 5

Printed in Canada

To my wonderful grandmother,
Stanka Ugenovic-Puharich

CONTENTS

ᴨᴨᴨᴨ

Preface   *1*

[1] In Chaos, There is Order   *5*
[2] A Brief History of Hospital Trains   *19*
[3] The Evolution of Hospital Trains   *37*
[4] The Trains of the Second World War   *51*
[5] The Nurses   *71*
[6] The Doctors   *83*
[7] The Patients   *93*
[8] The Battles   *105*
[9] The Future is Past   *121*
[10] The Secret Social   *131*
[11] The Image   *141*
[12] The Legacy   *157*

Acknowledgements   *165*
Notes   *167*
Bibliography   *183*
Index   *193*

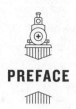

PREFACE

MY UNDERSTANDING OF HOSPITAL TRAINS came from my late grandmother, who was a nurse working on one during the Second World War. I say *nurse*, but in truth the nurses on those trains often had to act as doctors, surgeons, and even soldiers as the circumstances of war could make anyone into a polymath in a heartbeat. What takes years to learn and master in a controlled setting in times of peace becomes quick on-the-job training in war. The hospital trains were as transformative to patients as they were to the staff turning a moving train into a hospital amid gunfire, grenades, and bombs.

The idea of a moving hospital has always intrigued me. There are hospital ships, of course, but hospital trains had their own logic and ways, and for many, these trains meant the difference between life or death. Before reaching the ships, many patients had to be treated on trains.

Whenever I mention my grandmother's past life in conversation, I am surprised to hear how many people were born on those trains or had families who were rescued by them; many of those whom my grandmother saved made the trek to her house years after the war to thank her in person. They never forgot her, but the enigmatic sands of time often shift our attention elsewhere, and future generations are left unaware of the heroic deeds of the past. History is, of course, filled with stories, so I wished to chronicle an often-forgotten part of that war effort.

My grandmother saw her time on the trains as one of the happiest and most productive eras of her life. She shined brightest when she could be helpful in chaos as she survived and thrived and helped others do the same while bonding with her colleagues, who gave her, for the first time in her life, a sense of belonging. Tragically, when she returned home, she discovered that her entire family had been taken to concentration camps by fascists and murdered, including her youngest sister who was but a mere child. Yet, working on the trains had, in many ways, exposed her to people from all sides of the war, so she was able to put the tragedy in perspective and not turn bitter or bigoted in the aftermath.

I often think about what her life must have been like, how she thrived in the chaos of war, healing those who were destined to be destroyed by it; how she then floundered for years within the order that came with peace; how she lost her footing when restricted by the rules of a paternalistic society that forgot how brave and resilient women like her—healers and warriors—were when it counted the most. She not only took care of herself in war, but also others on the brink of death, often having to improvise when circumstances were uncertain and supplies were scant. And yet, after all that accomplishment, she ended up contained within the rote, limited role of housewife. I often wonder what the world lost when those women were whisked away after they arrived home, deprived of a true hero's welcome instead of being given opportunities to put their experience, vigilance, brilliance, and resilience to good use outside the home.

What did we lose when we made up societal rules that confined those who did their best when they were unleashed in the worst of circumstances? These were the healers who did not have to risk their lives for others; they could have easily plundered and harmed without fear of detection. Instead, they rose above the darkest circumstances and exemplified brilliance, altruism, and humanity.

The story of the hospital trains is not only historically important—it is also important to me personally because it speaks to the power of resourcefulness and perseverance, and it shows us ways of being to strive for in the world today. To those who braved the darkness to bring light, I dedicate this book and express my personal and eternal gratitude. May you, the reader, experience the same sense of wonder and gratitude by the end of the final page of this book.

One final note: this work is intended to be a gateway for those who know little or nothing about hospital trains. You will be introduced to them, their history, and their various incarnations in different nations, including Canada, as well as a discussion of the crucial role of women who worked on those trains. There is much secret history here, and though we have no shortage of brilliant, moving, and wonderful must-read books on the topic of the Second World War, the story of hospital trains has been largely ignored until now. Enjoy the ride.

1

IN CHAOS, THERE IS ORDER

ACCESS TO RAILROAD TRACKS DURING the Second World War meant the difference between defeat and victory, and life or death. It was often a wheel of fortune as much as it was a lifeline: your fate strictly depended on whether you reached the train in time, and what train came your way. War is always chaotic by nature; even a shrewd, cunning, and vigilant person can have providence work against the most ingenious of plans. As such, railroads were essential to stacking the odds in a society's favour under the worst and most unpredictable of circumstances.

Trains brought food, munitions, and salvation. They provided an escape, but many times they brought ruin and doom. Holocaust victims were sent to their deaths, and for some, the weapons were brought to their enemies to kill them. The wheels spun in every direction even as the tracks moved in a single line, yet there was one kind of train where the chances of survival greatly increased with its arrival: the hospital train.

Hospital trains were not new in the Second World War. Ambulance trains were employed in the Great War and evolved from there. In the First World War, there were twenty-one such trains in both the UK and France, operated by the American Expeditionary Forces or AEF. By the time the Second World War exploded, the UK had converted regular trains into moving emergency wards to tend to those critically wounded; it was an elegant solution as train cars could be refitted with tier beds and supplies could be easily transported along with medical staff.[1]

However, the psychological and emotional importance of the hospital trains, particularly in the Second World War, is often missed in our history books. We have all seen haunting images of genocide victims being boarded onto trains to meet their tortuous end in concentration camps. The various fascist factions, from the Nazis to the Ustaše, had institutionalized kidnapping innocents and thought nothing of sending their victims, including children, to slaughter. Whereas those trains brought certain death, the hospital trains brought life; the trains carrying innocent civilians to torture, starvation, and slaughter were symbols of chaos, while the hospital trains represented the order that brought people back from the brink of death with healing, care, and the latest medical equipment and medicine. These trains were as important as the troops who came to liberate and defend, and those who worked inside them bought soldiers and civilians alike enough time and space to survive and procure a victory.

Trains were not just equipped with healing staff, but also recreation workers; these workers, often overlooked, were called *pioneers* in news reports. It is interesting that what seems mundane now was considered newsworthy and prestigious in its time. For example, one such pioneer's daily schedule was published in the Saturday, October 14, 1944, edition of *The Fog Horn*:

Miss Helen Torkelsen, Red Cross Hospital Train Worker, is the pioneer in that field in this area. She is a resident of Salt Lake, and a graduate of the University of Utah. Was a commercial artist before enrolling for Red Cross Service. Her report on the first trip is given below—as she submitted it.

The Train Commander jumped gun! Train scheduled to leave at 11:30. I arrived at 11:00 to see last car easing out of Crissey Field ... into the fog. The hollow feeling I experienced reached down to my socks. Fortunately, a staff car was available, and I caught the train at 3rd and Townsend. The Red Cross was practically NOT at his side ... I was located in Car No. 2. First, all supplies were assembled neatly in the vestibule. I spoke with the Train Commander as to rest periods, lights out, etc. I was informed that I should be allowed to go into all cars at any hour of the day, until 9:30 p.m. ... lights out. I found that the patients were, for the most part, in excellent spirits, in proportion to their condition, and they thought Red Cross was really on the ball. I distributed cigarettes to all patients first thing in the morning, and after noon chow. I found it wise to leave a carton of matches with the corpsman in charge of each car, rather than to distribute matches to individuals.

Cards, maps, reading material and stationery were also distributed. Requests for comfort articles were filled during the morning. Slippers were in great demand, and my supply was gone almost immediately. It seemed wise to apportion reading material to each car for the day, and leave it with the corpsman in charge. This, supplemented by distribution of daily newspapers and current magazines, provided an adequate amount of reading matter. However, there is a great demand for current *Life*, *Time*, *Reader's Digest*, *Newsweek*, *Look*, *Click*, *Colliers* and *Sat. Eve. Post*. Westerns, comic books and national geographies of any date are popular. The supply must be varied to meet the tastes of individuals ... a major spent the entire five days improving his mind with the latest editions of Superman.[2]

Every facet of hospital trains was seen as newsworthy, from their manufacturing to their routes. Both news outlets and medical journals mused over them frequently. These trains were a symbol of power, survival, brilliance, compassion, and most importantly, the future.

Eventually, hospital trains fell out of favour after the war (though they are still in use in places such as India), but their quiet imprint on history cannot be ignored. The workers were the people who added more grains to the hourglass, ensuring that time would eventually favour order over chaos. From surgeries to amputations to delivering babies, the trains were about preserving life. While soldiers were forced to fight with every aspect of death in the chaos, the medical staff of the hospital train fought to find life in every nook and cranny they could find. Often, they were short-staffed, overworked, and undersupplied, yet they did their jobs. Amputations without anesthesia were performed, and frequently, but the result was still triumph.

The mobile hospital brought patients to conventional hospitals, and to other mobile hospitals such as ships, but delicate procedures were often performed en route, day or night, during calm and during battle. What needed to be done was done. There were secondary uses for the trains, including rescuing children who lost their parents through war or concentration camps, picking them up to take them to orphanages.

In modern times, we have become accustomed to the luxuries of peace, often taking them for granted, yet during the Second World War hospital trains were regarded with humility and gratitude. The healthcare staff on these trains did more than just heal the physically wounded: they also gave emotional and psychological comfort to the patients as well as the personnel.

Even then, the trains were a mobile hospital in every sense of the word, with contained dining areas, kitchens, offices, surgical cars, pharmacies, and sleeping quarters. They were revered in the press and were a sign of a nation's might as much as troop size and weaponry. The *Washington Evening Star* made a fuss on November 22, 1943:

> Washingtonians will have an opportunity this week to see the Army's first overseas-type hospital train, built especially for use in theatres of operation. The 10-car train, enroute to the California-Arizona maneuverer area for temporary training purposes, will be side-tracked for exhibition Thursday and Friday at the Fourteenth and Maine avenue yards S.W. . . .
>
> Known as the 3d Hospital Train, the unit consists of six ward cars, a kitchen car, utilities car

and two personnel cars for the staff of officers and enlisted men. It is of all-steel construction. Each car is slightly more than half the length of an ordinary American railroad car, so designed purposely to negotiate sharp turns, narrow bridges and tunnels of foreign railways. The train is olive drab in colour and displays all hospital and Red Cross markings in accordance with the Geneva Convention agreements.[3]

The *Evening Star* also had a piece on January 18, 1942, that was dedicated to the trains under the banner "The Noblest Act":

We had 262 on board and there was the smell of death in the carriages. I was sitting with Captain Benson, the conducting officer who showed me around at the front. We restrained an impulse to walk back through the cars and talk to the wounded. We had had enough war. We were, technically, on neutral soil now. There were big Red Crosses on our rooftops. The enemy would not bomb or strafe us here. The war was over for us, temporarily. For the men back there the war was over too, permanently.[4]

The article went on to describe why the trains became "neutral territory" during the war:

Some of the wounded were what you call "walking wounded." They weren't hurt badly enough to give them beds in the hospital cars. Our coach was half second-class compartments and half third-class lunches. The third-class half was filled with Italian and German prisoners. They were hungry too. You don't pamper the wounded on the trains. You shove them aboard and move them off. They get water and there's some thin soup for the bad cases, but the object is to get them to hospitals in Cairo and Alexandria.[5]

The *New York Times* in December 1943 touted in a headline, "Hope Reborn in Wounded As Hospital Train Goes West; Soldiers From Salerno, Sicily and Africa Quit East for Treatment Nearer Home at Yuletide and Aches Are Forgotten; HOPE IS BORN ANEW ON HOSPITAL TRAIN THE BEST WE HAVE IS HELD NONE TOO GOOD FOR THESE."[6]

News reports about the trains were common and described their varied uses. On home territory in the US, the trains were often used to give medical personnel practical experience before they were shipped off to foreign soil. Detailed articles, such as one in the *Washington Evening Star* on May 19, 1941, clearly illustrated for civilians the trains' intended uses:

The hospital car contains a kitchen capable of feeding 500 men at a single meal. It is also equipped with operating rooms for daily dressings, examinations and emergency operations. In addition, the unit car contains an administrative office for the entire train, quarters for two officers, a shower, and bunks for the kitchen personnel.

Each Pullman or chair car, which comprise the "wards" of the railway hospital, will be staffed by three Army nurses and three orderlies, working on an eight-hour shift. The nurses will occupy the drawing rooms at the ends of each car. An ordinary hospital train will consist of 10 to 15 cars and will be used in the ordinary course of duties to transport sick or injured soldiers to Army hospitals nearest their homes.

The car unit at Fort McPherson is the one that is now scheduled to take part in the summer manoeuvres in the "fighting" around Fort Jackson and Fort Bragg in the Carolinas. It is under the supervision of Col James E. Bayliss, 4th Coast Artillery surgeon.[7]

Hospital trains were an integral part of understanding the war. Their ubiquitous presence became an essential part of the war narrative, as it was in the *Lexington Advertiser* on May 3, 1945:

Among the patients aboard the hospital train to travel across the nation toward the hills and valleys of their homes was Pvt. John Shepherd, USMC, of Tchula. These boys were sailors and Marines who paid for the conquest of Iwo Jima and the Philippines with their limbs and their blood—three officers and 192 enlisted men. They boarded the Navy train on April 21st where they left the US Navy Hospital, Marc Island, Calif.

The men who had undergone amputations for an arm or a leg are being transferred to the US Naval Hospital, Philadelphia, Pa. It was the largest trainload of amputee combat casualties of its kind to leave the west coast, according to Captain A. G. Churchill, USNR, Twelfth Naval District Assistant Medical Officer, who with Navy doctors, Navy nurses and hospital corpsmen accompanied the trainload of men.

Two Red Cross welfare workers, the first to go aboard a Navy hospital train, took musical recordings, games and other recreational facilities to keep the men entertained as they made the long trek.[8]

Those locals who worked on the trains were often celebrated as heroes—for instance, the *Durant News* in Mississippi on July 6, 1944, had the headline: "Durant Boy Member of Hospital Train That Cares For Wounded

Soldiers: Capt. John B. Wilkes Transfers Wounded From Battle Action."[9] It was seen as a lofty honour to be in one, as the trains were a sign of technological wonder as well. As outlined in the January 1944 edition of the *Bulletin of the United States Army Medical Department*, the trains were planned to the meticulous last detail:

> A ten-car hospital train has recently been delivered to the Desert Training Center in California. It was furnished by the Transportation Corps in accordance with the requirements of the Medical Department. The manufacturer was Pullman-Standard Car Manufacturing Company, Worcester, Massachusetts.
>
> This train is made up of six ward cars, one utility car, one officer personnel car, one orderly car, and one kitchen, dining, and pharmacy car. Each car is 44 feet long, mounted on two four-wheel trucks. The usual vestibules at each end of the car are omitted and two wide doors, one in the centre of each side, are substituted to receive and discharge litter patients.
>
> The ward car provides eight two-tier bunks, sanitary service facilities, medicine cabinet, and an ash tray and water glass receptacle at each bunk. A folding support is included to hold a litter for emergency use. Folding seats are provided in front of the entrance doors for use when doors are closed.

The utility car is provided with two Vapor Clarkson Steam Generators, and two 15-KVA Diesel electric generators. A shower bath and locker space are also included.

The officer personnel car serves as living quarters for four officers at one end and six nurses at the other. Shower, toilet, and locker space are provided for each group. A writing desk, water cooler, and folding seats are available for general use at the center of the car.

The orderly car bunks are the same as those in the ward car. However, the centre area is provided with two toilets and lockers in lieu of the sanitary service facilities for patients.

The kitchen, dining, and pharmacy car combines a complete kitchen for the personnel and patients, dining table service for sixteen with two serving tables, and a small pharmacy complete with work table, sink, cabinets, and desk.[10]

The trains were built on the premise of order to make their way through the chaos, but often what is forgotten are those who fought to save lives in them as well as those who fought to live. They were an integral part of the war, and their depiction in the media was often moving and iconic to the very end as the *Los Angeles Daily News* recounted on June 25, 1945:

Gen. Dwight D. Eisenhower was delayed here 40 minutes today when a hospital train loaded with wounded servicemen passed through the small town station. Eisenhower learned that the hospital train filled with wounded soldiers all stretcher cases was just outside of town. As the train approached the station Eisenhower stood up in his jeep and faced the train. Grinning faces of wounded soldiers peered out of the long hospital train windows, looking for Ike. As they passed the general the soldiers gave him the thumbs up salute, and a few of the wounded men even managed a military salute. Eisenhower returned both salutes. Near the end of the train two army medical officers stood in an open door. The general asked, "How are they doing?" referring to the wounded men. "Very good, sir," the medics replied. The train pulled on through the Abilene station and Eisenhower boarded his special train for Washington.[11]

The trains were a central artery that gave hope and life, but once the Second World War drew to a close, the same majestic vehicles lost their rightful place in history. This book will explore how the hospital trains came to be, how they operated, their triumphs and tragedies, and most importantly, how they contributed to the restoration of peace, from Europe to Africa to North America. From their critical role in Dieppe to even their use in the US to evacuate soldiers from one hospital to another, these were the rides to salvation. While war is about fighting and using tactics through technology, cunning, and force, work on the hospital trains required different strategies that moved in the direction of peace. War is chaos, but even in chaos, there is order, and the hospital trains delivered that order in various ways until the end of the war.

Before we look at the psychological influence of trains on the war, let us begin by understanding the origins of the transportation that took passengers from chaos into order.

2

A BRIEF HISTORY OF HOSPITAL TRAINS

HOSPITAL TRAINS MADE THEIR MARK even before the First World War. In 1850, the Crimean War saw their debut; they were flawed in several regards, but as the trains were mainly used to bring supplies and equipment to the war front, it made sense to also use them to carry away the wounded on the trip back. As Michael Foley notes in his book *Britain's Railways in the Second World War*, what started as an afterthought began to form into its own concept:

> The use of hospital trains was not a new concept. They had been used in the First World War but had their origins in a much earlier time. The Grand Junction Railways had, as early 1837, a compartment in the mail van that could be converted to hold a bed for someone who was ill. There was a truck kept at Charing Cross that could carry a road

ambulance if needed, and by the outbreak of war, all the Big Four had a number of vehicles containing beds and all the necessities of the sick room.[1]

The concept of the hospital train was vital enough that it continued in various forms, improving over the years. They were also in use during the Franco-Austrian War, but rather than mobile hospitals, they were more so vehicles for transporting soldiers who were wounded or killed. These were not formally designed as places to carry out medical procedures but were the best and most efficient way at the time to bring the wounded to hospitals.

However, this is not to say that no one at the time had thought of adapting trains as medical facilities. Austrian physician Jaromir Baron von Mundy, credited as the father of Vienna's ambulance service, made a significant contribution to the evolution of hospital trains:

While Mundy was on an educational journey through England, the Austro-Prussian War broke out on 7 July, 1866. Mundy immediately contacted the Ministry of War to volunteer as a physician. He treated injured soldiers in the Battle of Koeniggraetz and supervised their transport to Vienna. The injured were bedded on straw and transported back to Vienna from the battlefield in cattle cars without any medical care at all. They were brought to the

Prater Park grounds, where a casualty clearing station had been set up under Mundy's supervision. Almost as many soldiers died during transport as on the battlefield. Mundy realized that the means of transport were unsatisfactory and racked his brains how to improve this intolerable situation. Thanks to his initiative, freight cars were equipped with shock-proof stretchers and the trains began carrying physicians and nursing personnel as care providers en route for injured soldiers.[2]

Mundy's foresight was evident, even if his colleagues at the time did not see it:

Moreover, Mundy worked on the constructing of stretchers, ambulances and giant spotlights for the transport of injured soldiers from the battlefield in the dark. Again and again, Mundy criticized the municipal medical aid in Vienna, because he believed that all patients transported from the scene of an accident should be accompanied by medical personnel and because there was no such thing as medical personnel trained to deal with potential disasters.[3]

Eventually, Mundy's warnings were heeded, but the process was a slow one. During both the American Civil

War and Franco-Prussian War, a similar setup was used to transport wounded soldiers. These were not the only campaigns to see a version of the hospital train that was used primarily to round up wounded troops to take them to more conventional hospitals.

However, by the time of the Spanish–American War of 1898, the trains had improved, though there were financial problems that nearly prevented their creation. The Kentucky hospital train took wounded soldiers during the conflict and had been a prominent staple in news reports. For example, on September 5, 1898, the *Maysville Evening Bulletin* reported that "the Kentucky hospital train left Chickamauga Saturday night with fifty-three sick men, most of whom belong to the Second Kentucky Infantry. In the number is Sam Colburn of Flemingsburg."[4]

Ohio had its own train, and like others, was reported on nightly. "The Ohio hospital train has arrived at camp. It will leave for Columbus with the sick Ohio volunteers as soon as possible."[5] The *Marysville Evening Bulletin* also made mention of a third train:

> The third hospital train sent here under the auspices of the Medico-Chirurgical hospital, arrived from Camp Meade, Pa., with more than 100 sick on board. Most of the men are suffering from typhoid fever.[6]

Although the daily reports of where trains went, how many wounded they transported, and their afflictions were common fodder for the press, the Kentucky train almost never came to be. The *Indianapolis Journal* explained on September 2, 1898:

> Governor Bradley will start the hospital trains to Chickamauga and Newport News to bring home the sick Kentucky soldiers at these camps on Saturday. After several banks had refused to loan the State the money necessary to equip the trains, the state treasury being empty, the Governor secured the necessary amount from the State National Bank at Frankfort. Dr. U. V. Williams will have charge of the train to Newport News, which will get the sick men in the Third Kentucky, while Dr. S. James will have charge of the train to Chickamauga, where the Second Kentucky is stationed. Four women physicians and nurses will go with each train, which will be provided with every comfort for the sick soldier boys.[7]

By December, the Kentucky train had served its purpose after a busy run and was retired, as the *Hope Pioneer* noted on December 8, 1898:

> A great improvement in the health of the army has taken place within the last two months, as

shown by the last reports to the surgeon general
from the held and general hospitals. The hospitals at Chickamauga Park have been emptied and
abandoned. The same is true of the division field
hospitals at Camp Hamilton, Lexington, Kentucky
and Jacksonville, Fla. The hospital train which
has carried nearly 4,000 sick men from the various camps to general hospitals is now lying idle at
Washington.[8]

The history of the hospital trains is one of slow evo-
lutionary progress. Although it wasn't until the Crimean
War that the notion of performing medical procedures
on the trains started to take root, each war had its own
unique set of conditions and realities, that contributed
to the development of hospital trains. As historian Alan
J. Hawk notes in the September 2002 issue of *Civil War
History*, the Civil War showed the potential of these
mobile units:

By allowing for rapid movement of the wounded,
the hospital train revolutionized military healthcare
by moving the patient to the physician, rather than
leaving the physician with the patient at the battlefield. These trains permitted the concentration of
patients at hospitals that could specialize according to the patient load and the physician's expertise,

foreshadowing the development of medical specialties that has become the hallmark of twentieth century medicine. In addition to the receiving better medical care, the patient's quality of life improved by allowing him to convalesce in large cities or near his hometown where his family could visit.[9]

The Russo–Japanese War (often dubbed World War Zero) also saw the use of hospital trains, as the July 16, 1904, edition of the *Globe and Mail* noted:

The correspondent of *The Times* at Kieff, under date of July 12, says: The twenty-sixth military hospital train, fitted out by the Ministry of War, has left Irkutsk. The whole of the Manchurian and Siberian Railway lines are systematically split into sections, and numbered hospital trains, replete with the best surgical and other appliances obtainable, are apportioned between these sections.

The staff of each train includes three or more doctors, six to ten nursing sisters of the Red Cross Society and thirty to forty hospital assistants. Each train has accommodation for from two hundred to three hundred wounded and sick. The hospital train was destined to run solely between Irkutsk and Kazan, where the hospital train and hospital steamer or barge services link up.[10]

Once the First World War exploded, the notion took off. Ambulance trains tended to injuries with their own personnel. Trains were associated with hospital ships, and the chain was well-established. Each had surgical wards and the supplies required to oversee proper medical treatments. The Great White Hospital Trains, as they were dubbed in the UK, made a difference in saving lives. The trains were common fodder for the press to discuss, usually with a local angle. As the January 7, 1915, edition of the Toronto *Globe* noted, who was on the trains was as important as the vehicles themselves:

> Lady Charles Ross, wife of Sir Charles Ross of Quebec, the manufacturer of the Ross rifle, is working in France on a hospital train which she equipped herself. Lady Ross was in Dunkirk when the German aviators dropped bombs on the town.[11]

However, those same trains also came under attack in the war zones. The *Globe and Mail* reported on March 9, 1917:

> Germany's uncivilized methods of warfare have been tabulated by the Russian Government. In a formal protest to the enemy Governments against violations of the usages of war, Russia enumerates the crimes of the Central powers, which have

resorted to the use of explosive bullets, gas, burn-
ing liquid, poisoned missiles, the poisoning of
wells, misuse of flags of truce and Red Cross flags,
killing the wounded, the bombing of hospital trains
and the sinking of hospital ships. Could savagery go
farther?[12]

There were tragedies as well. On December 27, 1914,
400 men were killed and another 500 wounded when a
troop train collided with a hospital train at Kalisz.

Despite this, the overall image of the trains was
associated with hope and optimism for the future. The
Tonopah Daily Bonanza, reporting from Fort Bliss, Texas,
on January 26, 1917, described in great detail the first US
hospital train to be put in service:

The new army hospital train, the first to be used
by the American army and the first in use on the
Western Hemisphere, recently took ninety-nine
patients from the United States army base hospital here to the general hospital at Hot Springs, Ark.
The train departed after having picked up sick soldiers at Nogales, Douglas, Columbus and other
army camps along the Mexican border. The train
is known officially as "Hospital Train No. 1, United
States Army Medical Department."[13]

The article gave a rare, detailed insight into the advances made in the train's design:

This hospital train consists of ten Pullman cars converted into wards, operating rooms, nurses' quarters and commissary department. Four of these have a capacity of twenty-eight patients each and two others of twelve patients each. The lower berths have been removed and white steel cots with steel springs put in their places. The upper berths were left but windows and doors were cut to give additional ventilation.[14]

But also, its visual aesthetic was a part of the article's fodder:

The operating rooms are furnished with white enamelled fixtures, the walls and ceilings are painted with white enamel and are as sanitary as those in a modern hospital. They are intended primarily for surgical dressing rooms. But an operation could be performed while the train was in motion.[15]

The large 200-patient capacity of the train was emphasized, but often, reporters were harder pressed to find factual information and used whatever little information they could glean themselves, as did one journalist in a June 8, 1918, article of the *Hanford Daily Journal*:

> This new American hospital train was built at the Dukinfield shops of the Great Central Railroad of England and will be shipped to the American forces. In France, it has every convenience for wounded men during transportation. There is a kitchen car and another for attendants. The letters "US" on the back show it is the property of the American government.[16]

Press reports at the time were content with describing just the outside lettering as it indicated national ownership, but as the simple system and methods improved after the Great War, so did the emphasis on more detailed news reports. The trains were well stocked, operated smoothly, and medical staff took better care of the personnel on board as technology and facilities advanced. As safe passage for the trains was more universally established, they not only accommodated wounded soldiers but now also included makeshift maternity wards.

The trains were also magnets for the West's most powerful and wealthy citizens, who were equally fascinated by them, as the *San Jose Mercury News* noted on February 15, 1916, when the US gave one to France:

A hospital train of thirteen cars, the gift of two wealthy Americans, was presented today by the French government. Laurence V. Benet, former member of the chamber of commerce in Paris, made the presentation address.

Justin Godart, undersecretary of state for sanitary service, accepted the gift. He referred to numerous similar acts of sympathy on the part of Americans and declared that their friendship for France was traditional.

The train is fitted with the most modern equipment and can accommodate 225 wounded persons.[17]

The event was prestigious enough to attract dignitaries and elites for the celebration, yet the underlying gravity of the trains' use wouldn't be diminished. By the time the Second World War began, the hospital train would finally come into its own and would become a triumph in technology and operation.

It was not just wealthy Americans who saw their potential. The trains gave women certain freedoms denied in more traditional venues. As Bennett noted in the *British Medical Journal* in 1992, Russian princess Vera Gedroits found a way during the Russo–Japanese War to practice surgery in a way that was denied to her under stationary settings:

After qualification Vera worked for a while in Professor Roux's clinic but did not settle, returning to Russia in 1900. In 1904 only 3.4% of Russian doctors were women. She published a variety of medical papers but because of her previous connections she came under the attention of the police (the dreaded Okhrana). Possibly because of this and from a sense of adventure she volunteered as a surgeon for a hospital train organised by the Red Cross. This supplemented the Russian army's medical department and was well supported by wealthy Russians, acting partly through altruism or possibly for the hope of some reward. The central committee was in St. Petersburg and under the patronage of the empress, who not only ensured that the staff was chosen from the city's best surgeons but also gave over rooms in the Winter Palace for sewing bandages.[18]

The arrangement, though dangerous, gave Gedroits the platform she required to do her work:

Among those who went to the Front in the service of the Red Cross as surgeons [was] the Princess Gedroits, chief surgeon of the hospital train furnished by the associated nobility of 40 Russian "governments," who was always at the front, operating in a specially constructed car, till the enemy's fire threatened the train.[19]

The train operators had practised and, throughout various wars, built on their systems: the availability of the trains allowed patients to be transferred to hospital ships and regular hospitals with little disruption. The Red Cross sign turned the trains into neutral territory, and less likely a target.

The reportage of the First World War was just a taste of what would be covered when the trains would reappear on the battlefield and in the press in later years. By the time the Second World War was in full swing, the trains were seen as a critical medical advancement, and their developments were discussed in detail in academic journals such as the *Delaware State Medical Journal*:

Forerunner of others to come, a ten-car hospital train for the United States Army Medical Corps has just been completed and is now in use for training purposes in Southern California before going to a combat area overseas.

The ten-car all-steel train was built at a cost of $135,000 by the Pullman-Standard Company and is illuminated throughout with fluorescent lamps in a variety of fixtures all specially designed and engineered by Sylvania Electric

Products, Inc., under special dispensation of the
War Production Board.

Staffed by five medical officers, seven nurses
and 33 enlisted men, the train is the last word in
modern equipment and design for the transport
of casualties. Narrower and shorter than stan-
dard-sized American railroad cars, the cars of the
hospital train were especially constructed to roll
on the sharp curves and steep inclines of foreign
tracks. Four cars are for personnel, 220-volt generators
and steam boilers for heating and ventilating,
kitchen-dining and pharmaceutical facilities.[20]

The journal went on to mention every aspect of this
brand-new wonder in medical technology:

Six of the cars are ward cars, each providing berths
for sixteen bed patients, or more "sit-up" patients
with the double-decker berths folded down. In the
centre of each ward car is an emergency operating area, a cleared space free of berths. Stretchers
may be carried into the train through double-size
doors in the centre of the car, placed on portable
standards, and used as an operating table without
transfer of the casualty.

At these points, as throughout the train, four-foot
fluorescent lamps, set in recessed ceiling reflectors,

furnish the illumination. Army specifications called for fluorescents for their advantages: they are cool, glareless and eliminate undesirable shadows. For the greater convenience of surgeons at work over a patient, and for the greater comfort of patients when the train is in hot climates, the Sylvania installation has been highly commended by medical men and the general public. The train made a series of stops for public inspection en route across the country from Boston.

From the lighting point of view, the train is apt to be a prototype for widespread post-war railroading.[21]

The trains were seen as cutting edge, which some of the biggest industrial companies attributed to their manufacturing. They were a symbol of a nation's strength and devotion to progress:

Sylvania was called in by Pullman, at the Worchester, Mass., plant and asked to do the job. Because the installation was for a train that was to be all-steel, an advantage at the battlefront, it was decided that the fluorescent fixtures should be steel. But about a year ago the WP asked all manufacturers to reduce the amount of metal in any single fluorescent fixture to the absolute minimum and Sylvania developed a fibre-type reflector. For the hospital train, however,

WPB cooperated and permitted steel construction. An exhaustive series of tests preceded the installation. Each of the different types of fixture[s] was put on a vibration machine, specially designed. The entire lighting fixture, including reflector, lamp, starter, sockets, ballast and wiring, was subjected to as many as a thousand rough vibrations per minute, varying from a sixteenth to a half-inch cycle. Only then was the apparatus okayed.[22]

Military medical supply catalogues included parts for these trains, such as guard windows, and much of the manufacturing revolved around making these parts safe and sturdy for the dangerous journeys around the most violent hotbeds of combat.

The trains were also seen as emblems of peace, and the press coverage about them often focused on those who survived over those who succumbed. As one December 1, 1918, *Washington Times* article recounted, the trains represented relief and escape:

Nine hundred American soldiers arrived here today from the German prison camp at Ullingen, by way of Switzerland. An American hospital train was awaiting the party, which comprised 700 officers and 200 orderlies. Their condition was unusually good, owing to the fact that food supplied to them by the American Red Cross actually had been delivered to them. In passing through Switzerland on their special train, the Americans were cordially greeted by the Swiss.[23]

By the time of the Second World War, from North America to Europe, the secret signal of might was in the development and efficiency of the hospital trains. Those who manufactured them were seen as a nation's might, while those who healed in the trains were the futuristic healers who were always on the move.

Reality would be a little less forgiving: there would always be issues with supplies and safety, and the stench of death was unnerving to both staff and patients alike— but as the next chapter explains, even these obstacles were overcome with ingenuity and innovation.

3

THE EVOLUTION OF HOSPITAL TRAINS

AS WE HAVE SEEN, HOSPITAL trains were by no means an invention of the Second World War; they had been in play for decades prior. By 1938, these vehicles would come into their own, but once the fate of the war was settled, the perception of trains shifted: Previously celebrated as a clever and efficient mode of providing essential medical access to peacetime civilians, they were now seen as old-fashioned symbols of the past.

The Second World War sparked innovation for trains as a mode of medical intervention, which is especially impressive given that they were like intricate, moving jigsaw puzzles that had to balance many needs. As author Clarence M. Smith noted in 1956, US-based trains overseas had many layers to them, and each layer served its own purpose:

[There] were two sets of three-tiered berths that could be used for seriously ill patients, for mental patients, or for medical attendants. This section was separated from the main ward by a sterilizer room on one side of the car and a toilet and washroom on the other. The main ward section had a row of five three-tiered Glennan-type berths on each side. They could be adjusted to provide seating space, or the two lower berths could be used for litter patients and the upper berth for ambulatory patients or attendants. Between the main ward and the vestibule were storage lockers and a shower bath on one side of the car, and a roomette each for an officer and a nurse on the other. Each car was carpeted, equipped with special lighting fixtures, and air-conditioned.[1]

Hospital trains could be categorized in several ways, but to continue our journey, let us look two specific categories: trains that were in operation during battles, and trains in countries that saw no combat on their own territory. It is interesting to note that those trains that saw no fighting still benefited from the innovations of those that did. Trains during this era would serve as prototypes for trains after the war was over. But how did the circumstances of war force the modifications of hospital trains? What was their significance during the war? To answer these questions, it is important to look at earlier wars and their own challenges.

We often forget that wars can spark their own set of solutions, as simple and obvious as they may seem in a modern world of hindsight. Railroad travel in the US began in 1827; by 1861, the US Civil War began, and trains would be modified to handle the changes in technology, landscape, warfare, and society. While this war inspired a sense of urgency to improve the trains' capabilities, the progress made was not always constant, and there were some gaps afterwards without major innovations:

> One innovation was the use of rubber slings to support the litters of the wounded to decrease bumping during transport. The trains carried red flags on the cars and the smokestacks of the locomotives were painted red to indicate priority handling and to indicate to the enemy the nature of the train. The next major American conflict was the Spanish–American War. No special cars were built or modified. A single train of parlor cars was used. The first real hospital train was put together for General John J. Pershing's Mexican Expedition in 1916. The cars were modified wooden parlor cars. Loading doors for litters were cut into the sides.[2]

Of course, along with progress came the possibility of accidents and disaster; those risks, and possible solutions to them, had to be factored into the equation.

On December 25, 1938, two passenger trains crashed in Bessarabia (today a part of Moldova and Ukraine); as the front page of the *Globe and Mail* reported the next morning, only another train could be equipped to deal with such mass carnage:

> Eighty persons were reported killed and 150 injured today in a collision of passenger trains in Bessarabia, south of Chisinau.
>
> With communications reduced because of the Christmas holiday, railway officials were unable to obtain details of the disaster immediately. They despatched special trains of doctors, nurses and salvaging equipment from Bucharest.[3]

In the First World War, trains were considered *ambulance* trains, as the mandate was to merely get the wounded and ill to a stationary hospital or unit. Belgium and France had a combined total of twenty-one of these cars and saw trains as a mere method of transport, with nurses from both the Red Cross and Queen Alexandra's (QA) Imperial Military Nursing Service on board to tend to the wounded until they reached the hospital. Author Nicola Tyrer describes the nurses' role in her book *Sisters in Arms: British Army Nurses Tell Their Story*:

QAs were involved at every stage of the operation, plying to and fro across the Channel to bring
home the wounded, and manning hospital trains in
Britain to ferry them on to proper medical care.
Because of the nature of the emergency, the vessels were not always hospital ships, but vessels of
all types hastily adapted to perform operations on
very sick men.[4]

Eventually, it dawned on those in charge that the
severely injured had a better chance of survival if arbi-
trary lines in the sand were ignored for reality and
pragmatism, and by the Second World War, the number
of hospital trains increased from twenty-one to thirty.

The US, like most other nations, had to start from
scratch. The ambulance trains of the First World War
were no longer viable, as Smith noted in 1956:

At the beginning of 1939, the Medical Department
had no hospital trains on hand and only indefinite
plans for procuring them in the event of war. The
Army had disposed of its World War I hospital cars
because it was cheaper to transport the few patients
who required movement in peacetime in Pullman
cars and tourist sleepers of regularly scheduled
trains.[5]

The means of turning trains into viable medical units was one of the many intricate puzzles to solve by the time Europe went to war again in 1938. How to best allocate resources and build a functional unit was no easy calculation under the circumstances. According to historian George H. Bennett, it all came down to the mathematics of the bottom line:

Breaking through the German defences would cost 25 percent of all the troops involved and a further 3 percent per day as the bridgehead was enlarged. Of the 25 percent initial casualties, 25 percent would be fatalities, 55 percent wounded, and a further 20 percent gassed. The threat of gas remained a constant worry for those planning for D-Day. Given that casualties would need evacuation and treatment, Allied planners were forced to come up with an assessment of the range of casualties that would need treatment. They determined that 43 percent would be stretcher cases and 57 percent would be classed as walking wounded. This would allow other planners to calculate the sea and airlift capacities necessary to deal with the problem of wounded. An evacuation plan involving aircraft, ships, mobile field hospitals, hospital trains, and hospitals in the United Kingdom could then be worked out.

This was one of many problems that the planners needed to address.[6]

How to build the trains would be only one of the many considerations; how to stock and maintain them would be another. In the UK, medical centres were kept in more rural areas, lest the German Luftwaffe attacked the wounded once again via an air raid. The mainline companies worked closely with the British Army, Navy, and Royal Air Force in this regard, converting regular trains into hospital trains as they were also tasked with supplying them under the watch of the Railway Executive Committee. Such undertakings began as nationally coordinated enterprises before becoming intercontinental and then global endeavours. Their common deficits spurred cooperation: necessity was the mother of invention for the Allies and became fertile, if often shaky, ground for collaboration.

Necessity is also the mother of re-invention: As casualties increased and cities came under siege, trains had to accommodate new problems with dwindling resources. Realities of the battleground led to modifications of the new trains. It was not only the mistakes from the First World War that were still fresh in the memories of engineers, the military, and various governments but the logistical problems of the ones in current circulation. For instance, escape routes had to be considered as well

as the kinds of rations that would be available. Author
Chester Wardlow noted in 1956:

> The Chief of Transportation also increased his con-
> trol over the utilization of Army hospital cars as the
> patient traffic became heavier. Because of his close
> contacts with the Surgeon General and the rail-
> roads, as well as his control over routings, he was
> able to avoid deadheading and other uneconomical
> practices much more effectively than the service
> commands. Consequently, early in 1944 the Chief
> of Transportation's Traffic Control Division began
> to assign hospital cars to specific movements,
> request railroad equipment for integration into
> hospital trains, establish schedules, and deter-
> mine what stopovers and diversions could be
> made en route. Similar supervision was exercised
> over the employment of the medical kitchen cars.
> In December 1943, with this increased control in
> prospect, the Passenger Branch had established an
> evacuation unit to deal exclusively with the move-
> ment of patients. This unit was responsible for
> advance planning as well as day-to-day operations.[7]

The Great War had seen trains as mere ambulances, but by the time the Second World War arrived,
the mobile hospitals now had kitchens, dining areas,

and even operating rooms, all of which required more supplies than their predecessors. Logistics would always have to be a key component in making the trains a successful undertaking, yet the full scope went beyond the stationary reality of the tracks and the battle lines. Both civilian and military nurses were recruited to work on the trains with the primary goal of getting the sick and wounded to another hospital: the traditional brick-and-mortar centres, but also the makeshift hospital ships. To appreciate the geographical logistics and mandates, we need not look further than the July 1949 edition of the journal *The Military Surgeon*:

> The plan agreed upon provided that Allied hospital ships were to bring German PW patients from the United States, Canada, the Middle East, North Africa, Italy, Northwest Europe and the United Kingdom to Marseille for transfer to hospital trains of both the United States Army and Swiss Railways for transportation to Bern, Switzerland, where allied PW patients from Germany would be exchanged. The trains would then return with the Allied patients to Marseille, transferring to hospital ships in the harbor, and would pick up a fresh load of German patients for transportation to Switzerland. The Allied hospital ships were to return to their native countries insofar as possible. Patients included Canadians, British, Americans, Indians,

North Africans, French, Australians, New Zealanders and French Indo-Chinese. This plan called for most careful timing all along the line. In execution, repatriates numbering close to seven thousand were duly exchanged, in a little over four days.[8]

A reassessment of the trains after being put into service in combat zones allowed governments to maximize their potential—a shrewd strategy given that nothing would be optimal. Supplies would be short. Space would be tight. Danger and desperation would be everywhere. Staff would be lost. By the latter half of the Second World War, the style and function of the trains had already been established and the routines were perfected. Some hospital train personnel relied on rations while others relied on farmers and even nature to feed them and their patients. Having to bribe gatekeepers was also a common practice to ensure the survival of both patients and personnel alike. Strategies were developed for designing the trains, but also for operating them.

But before getting to that stage of operation, particularly in the US, there were many disagreements among those in charge of the trains' construction:

After preliminary plans for the unit car had been drawn, the Medical Department Board and the Surgeon General's Office studied "in a new light" the Engineers' proposal to use only lightweight trains in theaters of operations. They found that the General Staff had "not specifically approved" the 20-ton car for a hospital train, but that it had approved (in 1931) the unit car. Moreover, they considered the train proposed by the Engineers to be "unsatisfactory" and "a reversion to that [type] used prior to 1863."[9]

A compromise was eventually met, paving the way for the evolution of the mobile hospital unit:

Finally, they had an alternative to offer: the unit car "included all the necessary facilities for the care of the sick and wounded" and could be used with commercial cars to make a complete hospital train either in the zone of interior or in theaters of operations. The Surgeon General and the Engineers then reached a compromise on 8 May 1940. The latter agreed with the Surgeon General that, as a first choice, hospital trains in theatres of operations should consist of the unit car and other heavy cars appropriate to it.

The Surgeon General agreed that hospital trains of lightweight cars could be used in areas where the construction of roadbeds made the use of heavier equipment impractical.[10]

When the trains were unveiled for public viewing, the show made headlines and drew crowds. The *Washington Evening Star* reported on one such event on November 25, 1943:

> Hundreds of women and a few men viewed the 10-car train today. In line with the Army drive for doctors and nurses, the District Red Cross set up a nurse recruitment centre in one of its mobile units, across the walk from the hospital train.
>
> Personnel of the train includes 4 medical officers (all doctors), 6 nurses and 33 enlisted specialists, trained in medical work. Nurses wore overseas seersucker uniforms.[11]

The display impressed audiences with its both its functionality and practicality:

> Observers were impressed by the completeness of the hospital unit. The 10-car outfit consists of six ward cars, each of which can accommodate 16 bed patients; a kitchen car, utilities car and two personnel cars for the detachment headed by Maj. Thomas Purser, Jr.
>
> Other features include a pressure ventilating system, complete sterilization units and emergency operating areas in each ward car.

This type of hospital train, officials said, is used principally to remove patients from evacuation hospitals, which usually are located within 25 to 50 miles of the frontlines, to the larger general hospitals several hundred miles to the rear. The olive drab train displays all hospital and Red Cross markings in accordance with the Geneva Convention agreements. Cost of the train, exclusive of equipment, was $135,000.[12]

While the finessing came in real-time, the net result was the creation of trains that facilitated healing and were designed to be as comfortable to the wounded as a train could be. Safety and shelter were priorities, and yet there would always be attempts to make the trains more comfortable and even cozy, far more than what even traditional hospitals could offer at the time. The notion of the *journey* was always part of the design, though the results were often mixed: the three-tiered bunks were made of wire and patients had little room to move, and trains often carried over three hundred patients at once. However, there were windows where soldiers could look out and see the places they were leaving behind. The evolution of the trains had a familiar theme: how to make the best out of a horribly catastrophic reality. The answers were never quite satisfactory, but they were good enough to give thousands the chance to see tomorrow.

[4]

THE TRAINS OF THE SECOND WORLD WAR

WHEN THE SHIFT FROM AMBULANCE trains to hospital trains occurred, it would prove to be a turning point in how medical treatment could be administered on a large scale. War inflicts not just injuries, but also infections, disease, and illness, and often all at the same time. Doctors and nurses, regardless of theatre, had to contend with the confines of reality, yet prove adept at manoeuvring and negotiating, whether by ground, by air, or by sea. Of the countless factors which dictated and defined how hospital trains were to be created, perhaps the most important one was centred around the need for evacuation. The train, despite being tethered to a track for moving, still had to be designed with escape and workflow in mind. The United States Army, European Theater of Operations unit, outlined key considerations for the trains in 1945:

Men with minor wounds often returned to duty from the evacs, but others requiring additional treatment and long convalescence were sent to Com Z general hospitals by trains and planes. After Paris was liberated, hospital trains became a vital link in the evacuation chain. These trains, almost complete hospitals within themselves, made runs from battlefronts to rear-line hospitals or evacuation ports.

Staffed by three officers, four nurses, and 35 enlisted men, the trains had their own emergency operating room and pharmacy. Seven or eight ward cars transported litter cases and one or two coaches handled walking wounded. A litter-type car accommodated 30 casualties, and an ambulatory car approximately 50.[1]

The concept of the hospital trains was simple enough to develop workable plans, but designing the cars had its challenges for other reasons: although the concept wasn't novel, its uses were small in scale, and there was limited feedback. There was little record of what was learned from trial and error—or *any* empirical testing—at the time as these trains were more of an idea in progress or an afterthought in the previous global conflict, as Clarence Smith notes:

> The convalescent hospitals and specialty centres, which became outstanding features of the World

War II hospital system, existed on a smaller scale
in World War I. The horse-drawn ambulance of the
Civil War gave way to the motor ambulance of the
two world wars, but hospital trains carried large
numbers of patients in 1864 as in 1918 and 1945.
Even the use of airplanes for transporting Army
patients in the United States, an important factor
in evacuation during World War II, had its small
beginnings in World War I.[2]

Smith also observes that there were limited options
available to the US military at the time:

Thereafter the Medical Department had assumed
that three types of trains would be used in the event
of another war: (1) trains made up entirely of government-owned cars; (2) "semipermanent" trains
composed of one government-owned administrative car, called a unit car, and an appropriate
number of commercial baggage cars, Pullman cars,
tourist sleepers, and chair cars; and (3) improvised
trains consisting of any available commercial rolling stock. Trains of the last type were considered
undesirable because they lacked accommodations
for the emergency treatment of patients and for
train administration. There were doubts that those
of the first type could be constructed in sufficient

numbers during wartime. Hence, emphasis was placed upon planning for the conversion of commercial cars into unit cars.[3]

Those limited options would be serviceable enough to create a functioning mobile hospital. The standard was fourteen cars, with each one having its own specific function. Supplies could be kept, the wounded could receive treatment, and everyone could sleep, move, and eat. Historian Larry Neal notes that there were three types of cars in the US Army's hospital trains:

> Ward cars, ward dressing cars (which included a small surgery area), and kitchen cars able to feed up to 500 people. These cars operated out of New York, New York; Hampton Roads, Virginia; Charleston, South Carolina; New Orleans, Louisiana; and San Francisco, California. The trains operated as one unit, with hospital cars moving from port to hospital. The train out of Hampton Roads often ran through North Carolina on its way to hospitals in Tennessee.[4]

The US model of the cars was designed to be functional and was built for a high volume of patients with the goal of saving millions of people. Nothing was wasted: neither time nor space. These trains were government designed and improved upon the deficiencies of the ambulance trains, as Smith asserts:

> [T]he unit car's kitchen facilities had helped to solve one of the major problems of World War I—the feeding of patients. Because of these advantages, and since the Engineers were already working on plans for cars for completely government-owned trains, the Surgeon General's Office concentrated in the winter of 1939–40 on the development of plans for an "ideal" unit car.[5]

The trajectory for the hospital trains would go in far more pragmatic directions. If the trains of the First World War seemed as if they were an afterthought, the new war would bring fresh opportunities to clear the slate and make the necessary leaps. However, centralized planning from the US Surgeon General's Office (SGO) had its limitations and often clashed with those in the private sector who dealt with the mundane realities of production up close, often causing friction and delays. Yet, despite this, progress and alterations in train design continued. Smith discusses these changes and how they became part of the first wave of the Second World War design in the US:

> The plans drawn were for a car that differed considerably from the unit car of World War I and to some

extent from one that had been planned in 1931. The latter presumably represented an improvement over the World War I car. It was to have side doors for loading patients and, in addition to the kitchen, an operating or dressing room and more space for attendants, but its capacity for patients had been reduced from twenty-eight to ten. In the fall of 1939, the Surgeon General's Plans and Training Division decided to eliminate all spaces for patients, in order to increase the feeding capacity of the kitchen to 500, enlarge the operating room and make an aisle around it, provide roomier quarters for more medical attendants, and furnish storage space for foods and medical supplies.

These changes were intended to produce a car which would have most of the facilities planned by the Engineers for the several administrative cars (dressing, kitchen, and personnel) of the proposed overseas train and would be "ideal" for use in mass evacuation in the United States.[6]

Interestingly, those same changes instigated by the SGO would not produce the desired results as the chaos and carnage of reality debunked the initial hypothesis of what was needed from a hospital train. An about-face by the SGO that reverted the trains back to a previous version of the train car eventually prompted a new theory in the design:

The surgeon general in charge of the US Army Medical Department wanted a return to the unit car design used during World War I. This style of car could handle the 30,000 wounded soldiers projected to return to the United States each month in 1944 and 1945.

Officials developed a new design in 1943, authorized it in 1944, and built it in 1945. Each of these new hospital unit cars included a full kitchen, a receiving area with side doors facing each other, a pharmacy area, room for 36 patients (including a six-bunk mental ward), two small rooms for doctors and nurses, a bathroom, and a sterilization room for medical instruments. The first order for one hundred cars was placed in late 1944, with delivery in early 1945. Another order of a hundred cars, numbered 89400–89499, was delivered between May and August 1945.[7]

By January 1942, the SGO decided the trains' designs had to be altered radically as the 1940 model had no space for patients, and serving food from one unit car to patients in others was difficult. Most interestingly, the soldiers riding on such trains in the US didn't require on-the-spot surgery, and the operating rooms were deemed to be too big and complicated to keep. On the other hand, the new trains would use air conditioning, something not factored into the first wave of trains; however, even this facet was not without bickering and controversy. The US-based trains, which would not be needed for combat conditions, were readjusted to make room for a different kind of design:

> To replace the unit car, the Surgeon General's Office and the Pullman Company developed a ward dressing car in the early months of 1942. It contained a small surgical dressing room and space for thirty litter patients, but it lacked kitchen facilities. It differed from the ward car only in the replacement of a toilet and berths for two patients with an operating or dressing room. This room, which could also be used as a loading room, was equipped with an operating or dressing table, a washstand, a sterilizer, and a locker for surgical instruments. The dressing table could be used in the centre of the room, moved down the aisle of the car to a patient's berth, or stored at the side of the car. Food would come from commercial dining cars.[8]

Versatility and minimalism replaced the original ideas of the trains:

> Instead of stationary Simmons beds, two-tiered Glennan adjustable berths were to be used in both

ward and ward dressing cars. Chief advantage of the latter was that upper berths could be pulled down to form backs for lower berths and thus make places for patients to sit.[9]

While the evolution of the US-based trains was always a work in progress, the ones destined to see combat in Europe would be constructed differently than the domestic ones; even then, some of the foreign-destined modifications seem almost trivial in nature, according to Smith:

At one end was a stainless-steel kitchen, with a refrigerator, an ice cream cabinet, a coal range, sinks, a steam table, and a coffee urn. Both the press and the Army called this the "principal innovation in the new car." Next to the kitchen was a pharmacy and receiving room, with wide doors on each side for loading litter patients. This room could be used also as an emergency operating or dressing room.[10]

As author R. Tourret explained in 1976, the hostpial trains were shilling not just coffee, but other treats as well:

Some hospital trains were produced by modifying FS coaches. The first was delivered for use on 21 November 1943, the second on 11 February 1944, and some more on 14 May 1944. The American Red Cross was supplying coffee and doughnuts by road, but to reach rail troops a FS coach was appropriately modified, including the installation of American doughnut machines, and then named "Yankee Dipper."[11]

Other changes were more important, particularly when it came to the original intent of moving away from the First World War models. As already mentioned, by the time of the Second World War, there would be radical redesigns and every part of the trains' construction was ultimately considered:

Planning for new trains began in 1939. The initial phase was the purchase of approximately 200 heavyweight parlor cars and Pullmans. Air conditioning was a requirement. The side doors for the receiving space were added. The regular passenger entrance was blanked off. Most of the cars had two levels of bunks for the wounded. There were Kitchen cars and the floor plan on the left shows a modified Pullman Mortuary car train with a kitchen on one end and an operating table on the other. This car had too many functions and few were built.[12]

By 1945, after years of tinkering, the train had became an engineering *Gesamtkunstwerk* —a total work of art—in which every piece of the puzzle finally found its place, according to Smith:

> The majority of the 1945 car order was built by American Car & Foundry in St. Charles, Missouri. The cars were of modern round roof configuration with riveted sides. The cars had individual kitchens at the brake end. They rode on 3-axle trucks. The internal configuration is similar to that of the converted heavyweights but with three levels of beds instead of two. The beds could all be folded up. The cars were to carry one doctor, two nurses and four service personnel. Up to 33 patients could be carried.[13]

Even if debates over coffee urns and ice cream storage somehow made their way to the design, the bottom line was maximizing patient capacity:

> Planning for these cars started in 1943 with the expected increased casualties from Europe in 1944 to be followed in 1945 by the Pacific casualties. 200 of these cars were built for use in the United States. 100 of these cars were retained in reserve.[14]

While the First World War's elites were less worried about the functionality of the ambulance trains, those in the Second World War often went the opposite route: there was often too much bickering over the smallest details at the expense of big-picture thinking. Eventually, reality would neutralize the disagreements, and the trains improved over time.

Even if there was heated debate within the halls of power, the public was not made aware of the exchanges. To the press of the era, they had not seen the problems nor asked about the discussions behind the scenes that shaped the trains' development. The concept of a hospital train was impressive enough, and for those whose lives were saved, they too didn't worry about those discussions, as survival and gratitude defined their thinking. When it came to civilian and journalistic reactions, the inclination was to praise the engineering brilliance of those who constructed the trains. The assumption was that everything was planned and those in charge held all the cards and knew what they were doing. Yet, there were instances when it was improvisation that impressed, as with one train in Algiers, reported on by the *Globe and Mail* on December 3, 1943:

> Working with discarded and bomb-damaged equipment, soldiers of the United States Army's railway service have constructed a L-car hospital train for use in evacuating wounded from the Italian front.

A company constructed the train in its spare time although the unit was operating on a 2-hour work schedule. The men searched bombed railway yards for usable pieces of equipment.[15]

If the US's designs were often secretly plagued by bureacratic clashes and a lack of focus, other nations had different experiences with their decisions over hospital trains. Canada's foray into hospital trains wouldn't arrive until near the latter half of the war, but when it arrived, it was seen as an emotional affair as feelings ran deep. The focus was on the train's ability to bring peace in chaos, and somehow, against all odds, turn the carnage into triumph. As one *Globe and Mail* article noted on November 29, 1943, the most important factor wasn't a victory, but the elation and relief brought by survival:

> Sombre skies, with a faint drizzle that flecked grey spots on white stretcher sheets, greeted Canada's first hospital train on its arrival at Exhibition Camp Saturday morning with 86 officers and men back from overseas.
>
> In sharp contrast to the previous night's stop at Montreal, where floodlights and surging crowds gave the scene a spectacular appearance, there was a grim-faced seriousness about the businesslike, though tender, speed with which Royal Canadian

Army Medical Corps personnel transferred stretcher after stretcher to waiting ambulances.[16]

The article went on to describe the emotional toll of the wait:

> And there was a tightness about the faces of the little groups of waiting relatives, a tenseness that seemed more vivid as the appearance of wide-grinning men brought sudden cheers, smiles or tears.
>
> Sharp to its slow-timed schedule, planned to avoid undue speed or car jostling, the hospital train slid gently to a stop at the embarkation siding in Exhibition Park at 9 a.m.[17]

The tight quarters could still accommodate spaces for medical treatment and living quarters.

Other nations had their own permutations and interpretations of what a hospital train represented. For instance, Canada and Australia had their own hospital trains, and each nation saw them through a different cultural lens. The Australian press's reaction to the lack of hospital trains was quick but pointed. It was seen as a scandal, as the *Adelaide News* noted in August 29, 1941:

> A hospital train for wounded men promised several months ago by the Army Minister (Mr. Spender),

following a disclosure that some wounded travelled second class without sleepers from Sydney to Brisbane, is not yet in commission. No official indication could be obtained today on when it is likely to be available.

Because of this, it is expected that some stretcher cases among six officers and 43 other ranks recently invalided back from the Middle East will have to remain in Sydney until fit to travel by ordinary train.[18]

Yet good, if short, news on the progress was reported in the *Barrier Miner* on February 5, 1942:

A hospital train of 11 cars, eight of which have been fitted with beds in three tiers, has been delivered to the military authorities by the N.S.W. Railways Department. It is the first train of its kind to be run on Australian railways during the present war.[19]

And on March 10, 1942, the *Adelaide News* made a vague and terse announcement:

Photographed at the Adelaide Railway Station on its first visit to this State. With large red crosses in white circles prominently displayed on the sides and roofs of carriages, it is fully staffed and equipped.[20]

The *Central Queensland Herald* had not much more to say about it in a March 19, 1942, piece:

> The first hospital train to be ran on an Australian railway in this war has been handed over to the Army by the N.S.W. Railways. Corporal McNally and Sergeant Ray are shown in stalling mattresses in one of the cars. A second hospital train has been assembled.[21]

Canadians had a warmer and more thoughtful regard for the national trains that brought soldiers home from war, although they were not designed to withstand combat. The focus was on transporting the wounded back home; and thus, it was public goodwill more than design that counted. A typical example of the framing comes from the *Lethbridge Herald* on January 6, 1944:

> With Mediterranean battlefields far behind and their home towns close ahead, the second large contingent of returning Canadian wounded are aboard this train today.
>
> Men who faced enemy fire and bitter enemy resistance in Sicily and Italy are lying in their cots and through the hospital car windows watching with almost unbelieving eyes the Canadian winter countryside—many of them for the first time

in four long years. This hospital train is carrying wounded and other war casualties to Quebec and Ontario only. A second hospital train is proceeding to Vancouver with casualties for the western provinces.

A brother of one of Canada's Dieppe heroes, Lt.-Col. C. I. Merritt, who won the Victoria Cross there, was among the wounded arriving at Halifax. He is Capt. F. W. I. Merritt, of the Seaforth Highlanders, from Vancouver, who received leg wounds in Sicily. He is aboard the coast-bound C.P.R. hospital train.[22]

The trains in Europe and in Africa, on the other hand, were the ones that needed to be designed for battle as much as for healing; they, too, were differentiated from their US, Canadian, and Australian counterparts, prioritizing efficiency and subsequently leveraging assets to create new lines of progress:

USA/TC hospital trains were obtained in the UK, probably because British coaches would fit any European loading gauge whereas American coaches would not necessarily do so. Coaches were converted for ambulance use at Swindon under USA/TC control. By 1 September 1943, there were 5 trains available and by D-Day 27. At the end of 1944, 25 of these trains were on the Continent, while some were still in the UK for use in the UK.[23]

In the UK, hospital trains were an organized and methodical affair, as the British Ministry of War Transport assembled thirty-nine trains for American use in the UK. While their medical equipment came from both the US and UK, these trains were entirely staffed by US medical personnel. According to the World War II US Medical Research Center, the British vulnerabilities were shored up with US resources:

[T]he shortage of material in the British Isles to construct rolling stock was a real obstacle. It was furthermore impractical to ship equipment and materials from the Zone of Interior as every available shipping space was at a premium and other priorities existed. The only solution came with the suggestion from the British Railways, that old passenger cars and diners be converted into hospital cars. British rolling stock could thus be used with the wagons altered by the (British) Swindon Railway Works according to specs (modified to fit existing British cars) submitted by the US medical authorities.[24]

A factor that affected how and where these units were constructed and employed was route planning, with considerations for the areas where enemies were likely to bomb or where extortionists were likely to obstruct the trains' paths. There would always be challenges and triumphs. Limited resources, and the painstaking calculations to optimize them, required foresight in how to best allocate the funds as well as considerations on how more resources could be gathered to make up for the depleted supplies. France put a 1500-franc toll on their railways, making hospital trains pay for the privilege of saving lives.

Yet all major European nations had their own version of the trains, with particular note to the UK who had managed to walk some fine lines and leverage what they could, as Tourret notes:

> Forty hospital trains served the US forces on the Continent, 25 of British origin, 14 of French material and one American (experimental). British ambulance trains went to Dieppe and Ostend. From September 1944, these trains had worked from Hasselt via Brussels to Amiens. When the Seine bridge opened in September, they then worked through to Bayeux.[25]

On the other hand, French railways, once the best in Europe, quickly fell to German forces. While France had ambulance trains during the First World War, their rail lines were now occupied by the Germans, who used them to loot an occupied France while carrying out Jews to their deaths in concentration camps. The UK–US alliance, on the other hand, made up for the void on the French railways. There was no doubt that the trains alone could greatly reduce the number of deaths, but having medical staff aboard those units who were able to perform tasks with minimal impediment could turn fortunes around.

The war proved that the trains could work and deliver when they arrived. Their construction was sound and elegant enough to do the job for the thousands of soldiers and civilians who were fortunate enough to be rescued and evacuated with them. However, no matter how well they were designed, it would not have functioned as successfully unless the personnel on board had the skills and savvy to make the most of them.

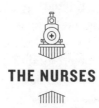

THE NURSES

IF THERE IS A SINGLE misconception surrounding the Second World War that permeates through the ages, it is that it was a war fought by men. Women were not labelled soldiers, but they fought on the battlefields as nurses, with their work overturning death sentences decreed by gunfire, grenade, or bomb. Nurses could be found in traditional hospitals, transport planes, and hospital ships, but the ones who zigzagged throughout Europe were the ones on the trains. In many ways, they were more than just nurses—they were also ambassadors for a future based on peace and healing. In many other ways, the nurses represented the future in a dismal present that had imploded from the ineptitude of the past. During a bleak time that hinted at a grim and hopeless future, nurses did more than heal bodies: they recalibrated souls to remind the wounded that the future was not a foregone conclusion.

While nurses, regardless of venue, represented that quiet visionary future, the ones on the hospital trains were often the first sign of hope the wounded would encounter on their way to being restored.

Even more intriguing is how many young women of the era worked in factories, as reflected in the iconic image of Rosie the Riveter; some of those women helped to build the very ships and trains the nurses travelled in to heal the sick and the wounded. Both sides of the equation are rarely connected as a cyclical unit of life in the history books and documentaries chronicling the era. Many more young women worked on the railways, which proved to be a lifeline as well. Women kept the cycle of life going, even when there was nothing but horror, fear, suffering, and death.

While it is easy to gloss over this singular trinity, it is important to focus on how hospital trains facilitated this vital nexus of life. From this triad, it was the nurses who were the face of the future: they were the ones who tended wounds, cleaned, fed, listened to, and touched the broken and wounded in close quarters. They travelled from one place to the next, dealing with hundreds of patients at once, yet left more than just an impression on them: they reminded the injured and ill alike that their lives mattered and their fortunes could turn. While doctors were one part of the equation, nurses took a more direct and hands-on role in the recovery journey.

No prior war had nurses working so close to the front lines as they did in the Second World War, mostly because of the mobility they had via hospital trains. British artist Evelyn Mary Dunbar, who made her mark portraying women at work during the conflict, immortalized hospital nurses in a 1942 oil painting simply titled *Hospital Train*. Yet the near-empty car and peaceful scene gives little hint of a typical day for those in such circumstances.

Nurses were also responsible for ensuring relatively low death rates among the injured: for instance, fewer than 4 percent of US soldiers who received medical care in the field or were evacuated died from wounds or disease. Much of that success comes from the triumph of the trains, which allowed the earliest possible medical intervention and enabled patients to socialize with others who shared the same traumas.

However, the idealized image of nurses often glosses over their true contributions. Many nurses, particularly from eastern European nations, had to defend the trains from hostile forces and needed to operate a rifle when essential. When there were heavy casualties and doctors were overwhelmed, nurses quietly had to take on medical duties beyond their own professional titles. The notion of separate and mutually exclusive roles in times of chaos didn't always translate so easily in reality, particularly for the nurses who worked on the trains where improvision was often required to navigate out of tight spaces when the chips were down. The railway lines often blurred the lines, not just for nurses, but for doctors who often had to resort to bribery to ensure supply lines remained open.

Often overlooked is the extent of a mobilized global force of nurses who congregated in the world's most dangerous places. Both Canadian military nurses—also known as the Nursing Sisters or Bluebirds—and civilian ones had been a familiar presence in Europe and were ready to heed the call to the frontlines. In fact, so many young women volunteered that there was a freeze on volunteers a mere ten days after the initial call. Many Canadian nurses joined British, US, and other nations' nursing efforts in Europe. Those who stayed in Canada often worked on the domestic hospital trains that brought wounded soldiers back home, while the nurses who opted to work overseas made their way on the trains of the nations they were posted in. For many of the wounded, this would be the first time they would come face to face with someone from outside Europe's borders, either being treated by a Canadian nurse or an American one; for many of these nurses, this would be the first time they ventured out of their own nation's borders to travel through Europe.

Because of the stakes and the dangers, few nurses could rely on predictable routines. Competence came from direct experience, and even then, there was always some spanner in the works to overcome. Some nurses broke under pressure, but the majority made it through, though some had trouble accepting their own limits, regardless of their impressive results. Author Kathi Jackson notes:

> So much publicity was given to the combat nurses that women who couldn't meet the criteria sometimes felt inferior, but they shouldn't have because their services were desperately needed in all the veterans' hospitals, debarkation stations, military bases, hospital trains, and air transports within the United States (also known as the Zone of Interior) and its chain of minor theatres.[1]

Hospital train nurses had to be the most versatile and cognitively agile: they were the ones closest to combat and were always on the move, travelling from place to place, picking up the fallen and healing them en route to a larger and more stable hospital, all amid air raids and gunfire. A red cross emblazoned on the train's exterior was supposed to provide assurance that armies wouldn't attack, but between playing dirty and collateral damages, it was no guarantee. Situations would change rapidly, and no one really knew what to expect looking out the windows. It was always a game of roulette inside the trains, as well as outside. Nurses needed to navigate through both worlds on an ongoing basis.

Nurses on trains came from most European countries and from North America. There could be language barriers and culture shock, yet it was not just in Europe where Canadian nurses could be found. As historian Cynthia Toman notes, nurses from the True North could be found in every major medical venue in Allied territory during the war:

> The Canadian Nursing Sisters were posted to all of the major theatres (the United Kingdom, Northwest Europe, the Mediterranean, and Hong Kong) as well as to military hospitals across Canada and in Newfoundland, the United States, and South Africa. Besides serving in diverse geographical areas, they also worked in different types of medical and surgical settings: military hospitals, prisoner of war and internment camps, specialty hospitals, casualty clearing stations, advanced surgical units, field dressing stations, field surgical units, hospital ships, and hospital trains.[2]

Regardless of where the nurses came from, the trains were highly functional units, largely thanks to those who ensured the trains fulfilled the mandate of healing and safe passage. Despite the chaos, order had to be established to ensure both patient survival as well as the survival of those who looked after them. The trains were the backbone of establishing a helpful rhythm. As the *American Journal of Nursing* noted in its June 1943 issue, despite the relative novelty of the venue, the tasks nurses needed to perform would be familiar:

> Each ward car has space for thirty-two bed patients in double-deck beds.
>
> A dining car with a kitchen provides for serving meals for patients and medical personnel and another unit car has a completely equipped dressing room. There is a baggage car for equipment and Pullman cars provide berths for the personnel.
>
> Either five or six nurses are assigned to each train, according to the request of the commanding officer. The nurses' duties and responsibilities are much the same as those of nurses in a hospital—to keep the patients clean and comfortable, have their meals and treatments done as ordered by the physician. The difference lies in the surroundings in which these duties are performed.[3]

As hospital trains could be found in almost all parts of Europe—from the west to the centre to the east cultural differences had to be taken into consideration. Despite a romanticized notion of trains and meaningful sacrifice, the reality for nurses on trains was always frustrating. Patients were edgy, in pain, and uncertain of their futures. Nurses had little time to reflect or indulge in self-care, and subsisted on rations or were forced to forage for food. As Diane Burke Fessler recounts in her book, *No Time for Fear: Voices of American Military Nurses in World War II*, nurses had to offer strong shoulders for patients even in the worst of times:

> Our drinking water was from a lister bag, and puri-fication tablets were dissolved in it, which made it taste strongly of chlorine. We were allowed one canteen of water each day and added lemon crys-tals from our K rations to help with the taste. We usually ate K rations, which were small carboard boxes filled with hardtack crackers, a tin of either cheese spread or potted meat, a fruit bar made usu-ally of ground raisins (or on rare occasions, ground dates), an envelope of lemon crystals, and enve-lopes of powdered coffee and sugar.[4]

Yet the K rations were far more appetizing than the lower grade ones, as the US nurse recalls:

> Sometimes we had the dreaded D rations ... [which] were only thick, heavy, sweet and strong chocolate bars, loaded with vitamins. If you gagged just trying to eat them, you could always dissolve them in hot water and have hot chocolate.[5]

However, the rations for US nurses were a luxury compared to the trains with European personnel who often had to forage for apples or tomatoes in fields. If some farmer had something to spare, there would be cornmeal to eat. The Red Cross would drop supplies from airplanes and many of those who worked on the trains could gather vital resources that way; some nurses would use the fabric from the parachutes to make clothing for themselves and others. Nothing would be wasted.

While nurses were the ones who turned fortunes around for many people, it is often difficult to find records of their post-war recollections of their time on the trains. One article in the *Progress-Index* of Petersburg, Virginia, on September 8, 2016, profiled a nurse's time on the train decades after her service:

> While we honour those who serve, sometimes we sometimes overlook the heroes who served them in turn. Were it not for scores of nurses, both on the front lines and at home, many soldiers may never have made it home.
>
> Elizabeth "Liz" Piecek was one of those nurses during World War II, serving on hospital trains that took wounded soldiers back home or as close to home as those trains could get them.[6]

Piecek's task wasn't just to be a nurse, but often also a therapist to soldiers who were on the edge and terrified:

Piecek recalled one of her first patients from one of those trains.

"He was a little fellow and told me, 'I don't think I will make it home to Utah.' I told him, 'Yes you are going to make it home!'" said Piecek. "He knew I wasn't going to accept anything else, and he did."

He was far from the only one who Piecek saved in her time on those trains.[7]

Despite her talents, though, she didn't wish to continue the journey when it was time to leave:

One week away from her three-year expiration of duty she was told that if she stayed longer than one week she would be promoted to captain. Her response was a typical one for any veteran.

"I told them 'Keep your railroad tracks, I'm going home!'" said Piecek.[8]

It is clear that the roles of nurses on these trains were ever-changing, and the definition of what a nurse was expected to do shifted depending on the circumstances of the time and place. The focus was exclusively on survival, requiring chameleon-like abilities to shift from role to role. The meta-role of a nurse was exhausting, and despite the victories and breakthroughs, burnout was frequent.

After all, the trains, despite agreements that no side in the war would attack them, were always in peril. Danger was always a factor. While UK hospitals shrewdly retreated to rural areas to escape the air raids, those on the trains were always a moving target. Nurses had to keep cool and assure the patients while helping to heal them. As author Eric Taylor notes:

> They had just stopped at the site of another casualty clearing station and were about to unpack when orders came for them to move everyone to the nearby railway station as quickly as possible. German infantry were close at hand. Once there they waited over an hour for the hospital train; shells rained down all around them. With the enemy barely twenty minutes away the train arrived and everyone got away to Number 50 CCS, where nurses immediately started attending patients again. "The first day I fed the operating theatres and kept the tables going with dressings and gloves. Men seemed just to pour in. Surgeons and the Matron were simply splendid. They worked with the rest of the staff day and night. There was no time for regular meals or sleep," recalled Sister G. Wicker.[9]

Despite the questionable supply lines and the gunfire, the nurses on the trains delivered: trains often had the stench of sickness or death, and patients often suffered without medication, but the nurses persevered despite the odds. The goal was to get the sick and wounded to a safer hospital, and in that, it was a triumph. Many casualties who survived could do so thanks to the trains—and because of the nurses who worked tirelessly in tight, suffocating quarters, with very little rations to keep themselves going, and without fuss or expectation of recognition.

[6]

THE DOCTORS

IF NURSES WERE THE UNOFFICIAL ambassadors of the hospital trains, then the doctors were the secret negotiators who had to do far more than administer medicine to ensure patient survival. Because space and resources were limited, the decisions doctors had to make were always high stakes, from how to operate on patients without anesthesia to how far to push when using novel methods to save lives. There were limited funds, limited supplies, and limited staff, yet the trains still saved millions of civilians and soldiers alike. Often, doctors had to resort to threats, bribery, and other forms of down-and-dirty methods to minimize death.

The trains on the battlefield took the most severely wounded, meaning there was always urgency. The trains in non-combatant nations took the walking wounded home. It was up to the doctors to make judgment calls and devise strategies to get those dying out of the clutches of death and then get them home. It was a tall order, yet any post-mortem of hospital trains almost exclusively became a discussion on the nurses, not the doctors.

Historical records provide a fascinating look at what was done beyond medical care. German prisoners of war, for instance, were tasked with unloading the wounded off the trains per doctors' orders. No resource or opportunity could be wasted, and often, doctors had to find creative ways of leveraging the smallest of breaks in the fighting when they had no cards to play, including relying on enemy soldiers to carry the very people they wounded.

Unlike other physicians who worked in traditional hospitals, or on hospital ships or planes, hospital train doctors had to move from town to town, country to country. They had to contend with a variety of unpredictable obstacles, and were, in many ways, professional transients. They managed to perform impossible tasks, and it often took creative thinking and darker impulses to get the job done.

Yet the performance of the doctors amid the fighting was seen as impeccable by those who were saved by it. Doctors were not mentioned by name, but by deed. Such was an example in the November 27, 1943, edition of the *Globe and Mail*:

> Take it on the authority of the men who faced death in Sicily, the Canadian Army Medical Services are equal to the best anywhere.

Soldiers aboard the hospital train that arrived here tonight told stories of men being operated on in the front lines almost immediately after being wounded, and they say that no matter how far forward the troops penetrate, the medicos are right with them.

One officer said, "It's a God-given right to grumble," but that he never heard a complaint about the medical services in Sicily and Africa.[1]

The speed and efficiency of operations and treatments defined the train physicians at every turn: in Europe, Africa, and North America. Stress was high, but few doctors worried about plaudits or recognition, regardless if the train rode in war or peace. As author William Feasby notes, decisions needed to be made immediately to be treated before problems became a crisis:

On one occasion in conjunction with the sick bay a hospital train was organized at very short notice to bring stretcher cases—all of whom were suffering from immersion foot—from Liverpool, N.S., to Halifax and for this both medical and nursing personnel were provided by St. John units.[2]

Doctors had no time to reflect, but instead had to react to situations on the fly while contending with a small staff and limited resources. Often it was the nurses who had to take up doctors' duties, performing amputations on soldiers, with or without anesthesia, or stitching up wounds when more doctors were required than what the train could carry, especially when the time was too short or distance too long to wait for treatment to begin after transferring the patients to a ship or building. Trains had limited capacity, but casualties were plentiful. These gambits were employed silently, but it was a judgment call between following the rules or navigating and negotiating with reality.

Alterations in treatment were necessitated by the confined spaces on the trains:

> Fractures of the humerus were usually immobilized in a shoulder spica with the arm down and forward across the chest so as not to obstruct the aisle of a crowded hospital train, plane or ship and not to bump against an overhanging bunk or stretcher. Special apparatus and equipment were frequently lacking in these forward installations and shoulder spicas were commonly applied with the patient's back, shoulders and head supported on a broomstick placed longitudinally on the table or stretcher beneath his spine. A modified Goldwaite frame, however, could easily be improvised and it facilitated the procedure considerably.[3]

While the public image of trains was often presented as well-oiled mechanisms with clean linens and well-stocked medical supplies, the reality was that they were operating on shaky supplies depending on the number of casualties, and as mechanical breakdowns were frequent, trains often failed in the middle of intense battles. Then there was the matter of making up the deficits in efficiency. The results were not always on the level, as one doctor recounted in 1983 (translated from Hungarian):

> Between 1942 and 1943, No. 111 on a hospital train I was an assigned surgeon. After the summer bridgehead battles with the eastern occupying group, then the winter one in connection with the ... disaster, I lived through the army's death march with a fragment of the 2nd Hungarian army. 1944—between 45 and 107 the 2nd reserve on the hospital train assigned to the corps, I served as a reassigned surgeon and was part of a series of retreats from the Berezina ... all the way to Denmark.[4]

He went on to describe the emotional prelude that placed the train in such a precarious position:

> In August 1942, the many dead and Korotojak and Urivi bridgehead battles following the wounded, in which our health posts, our field hospitals, they

worked day and night. The hospital trains also with a full load, they made their way through many dangers . . .

After Novi-Oszkol, he also loaded in Sztarij-Oszkol. This there were a lot of flies at the station of the latter place, and the during loading of wounded through an open window the flies in such swarms overwhelmed the white car ceiling, as if with a continuous black sheet would have involved them. A scary sight. Fly swatter we didn't have the material. However, as the train sped up, the strong air train came to our aid, sweeping the flies out of the cars through the open window.

We breathed a sigh of relief.

But then he got a surprise.[5]

The surprise in this case was an outbreak of gangrene, which was undoing the progress doctors had made only a short time before:

I opened the wound and covered it with gas edema serum I injected full. Bringing the patient out of shock it didn't work, he died within half an hour.

Our train in the area of Kursk at night torn apart. During this time, as it is running out our gas edema serum needed to be replenished, I managed to get 10 vials of gas edema serum . . .[6]

How the doctor restocked the supplies required a street-smart mindset:

It was not enough the Kursk train wreck, but also near Kiev, he also had the misfortune that the Kiev railway bridge was damaged by the partisans, and until it is restored Darnica, Kiev, director of Transdnieper . . . [We] bribed at the train station. Another three during this time gas gangrene developed, these are also the wounded in connection with massive shrapnel injuries to his muscles. I have used quite a lot of gas edema serum without any results. I asked the Kiev field hospital for help by phone. The surgeons who came out air injection was attempted around the wound done with deep incisions, but this until unloading we lost all three patients.[7]

Yet the results meant the job got done, and despite the trauma, it was an era he enjoyed since he triumphed over death and despair:

I will write my memories. Among the large group of wounded, there was always someone under the bandages who gave personal information about what happened to them. . . . [My] friends who are doctors, veterinarians, and team officers who are still alive told me from their personal experiences events that have not yet been included .... World War II was not explored in domestic literature. Even if the memories have faded a little, it would be a shame to leave them in the shadows of oblivion, even if one day they become mere data in the history of Hondvédek.[8]

Doctors had to work against grim odds, and because of this many physicians kept a low profile when interacting with patients. Nurses, on the other hand, spent the most time with patients and were remembered fondly. The doctors stayed in the background and often went against their natural inclinations to connect socially. The nurses became emotional savants while the doctors became primal ones. Together, they became an unstoppable force that bought patients time before they reached the main hospital on the ground or at sea—despite the constant fear of defeat and the walls closing in. Soldiers had one set of battles, but doctors had several. They were the soldiers without weapons, only tools to heal. The sky could fall at any second, yet despair was not an option:

The opportunity of evacuating cases to a hospital at the base so that they could receive treatment there rapidly ceased. Disorganisation of evacuation facilities set in at an early date. Roads were blocked by transport and columns of refugees and strafed by aircraft. Ambulances could not get through and as often as not were themselves the objects of attack from the air, in spite of the Geneva red crosses painted on their roofs. Within a few days evacuation by train had ceased. Some hospital trains had run into stations only to find they were occupied by the Germans; others were rendered useless by the destruction of the railway tracks. Evacuation of patients would be planned, only to be cancelled at the last minute, and in time ceased altogether.[9]

While hospital trains saved thousands, directly and indirectly, it is most peculiar how out of all of the players, it was not the doctors who captured the imagination of the public or the press. There were fewer per train, and they did not have as much to do with the social and emotional aspects of patient care as the nurses did. It was a near-anonymous task, but without them, a much darker outcome would have occurred.

THE PATIENTS

THE IMPETUS OF THE HOSPITAL trains was the patients: they were the most important factor and the prime consideration. They were the most vulnerable and the ones with the least power. Where they could go and what they could do was dictated not just by medical staff or military personnel, but by the confines of illness, injury, psychological trauma, and gunfire. Wounded soldiers needed to be stitched up, while civilians who, if they didn't become cannon fodder, were at risk for infection or disease. Some soldiers had serious psychological traumas and were a danger to themselves or others. The newspaper narrative romanticized hospital trains, but the reality wasn't always so noble. Optics were important during the war—too many fatalities and too little hope would mean that the morale of both the troops and the populace would vanish, giving the enemy a chance at victory. It was essential that faith in the system and the rules was never shattered. The hospital trains not only saved lives but sent a message to the public that neither the military nor the government would ignore their suffering or imperil them; it was a delicate and tacit balance.

From soldiers to infants, those who were taken into hospital trains from various battles were offered a lifeline. While hospital ships, planes, and traditional venues also saved many more by their sheer capacity and staff, even those positive outcomes came from the critical intervention of hospital trains during combat, disasters, and other potentially fatal circumstances. After gunfire, bombs, and outbreaks, the trains picked up the fallen and wounded, whether allies or enemies. Where there were divisions outside of the trains, inside there was collaboration.

Once soldiers were deemed too wounded to return to battle, they would be sent away by ship or plane before taking one more journey by train back home. The trains ran around the world, and for years as the war raged on, somewhere around the world, there was a train carrying the wounded to another hospital or to the loving arms of families back home. In nations such as Canada and the US, civilians saw hospitals as places where loved ones would be restored to their lives; North Americans also regarded hospital trains in an emotional light that differed from the perspective in Europe. A typical article describing these trains was presented in the December 13, 1943, edition of the *Oakland Tribune*:

> The long road back home to thousands of American boys who have been maimed for life has been smoothed, cleansed and made as comfortable as possible by the Army Service Forces.
>
> As a guest of the Army's second service command, I have just spent three days aboard a swanky hospital train carrying the armless and legless, the blind and the partially insane from Halloran General Hospital in Staten Island to Fletcher General Hospital in Cambridge, O.
>
> To the relatives of the victims, I am able to say that they are receiving the best care that American medical science has devised.
>
> The Army invited the press on this grim voyage to allow us to see how well these boys are cared for after they become battle casualties.[1]

Because the entire impetus for the trains was to reduce the number of deaths while keeping morale and faith unbroken, the trains were in some part theatre. It meant that how patients were treated on the way to the permanent hospital was carefully considered and tacit strategies were developed. Doctors healed, but it was up to the nurses to provide bedside manner: the human touch was considered an implicit but essential part of the job. Soldiers were encouraged to socialize, and they were engaged. Despite the injuries, the goal was to keep patient morale as high as possible.

It was a daunting expectation as the nature of the injuries of those in the trains was often severe, since it was often the most dangerously vulnerable who were boarded into the trains. The term to describe many soldiers was the *walking wounded:* these were the men who could move and function, yet were usually missing limbs or eyes. These injuries would now serve as a constant reminder of the trauma for those who made it out alive, yet they were the lucky ones who made it home and could function. Others became permanently disabled, either suffering from permanent brain damage or losing limbs, one of the most common the soldiers' injuries of the war.

In either case, regardless of disease or injury, most times, the walking wounded would be kept in separate cars or even trains. Fighting disease, infections, and outbreaks was a more complicated and difficult task, especially as many essential tools to prevent a lethal outcome, such as disinfectants and antibiotics, were in short supply. Operating tools could not always be properly sterilized, and when trains often had 200–300 patients on board, it was important to keep the walking wounded away from disease to minimize the body count.

But for those who suffered more severe injuries, there were always new dangers presented in hospital trains. Too many patients and a shortage of staff and resources could lead to new injuries or complications. The caregivers treating those who had become helpless could see the limitations and dilemmas of transient care, as Canadian neurosurgeon E. Harry Botterell and his colleagues discussed in their groundbreaking work on paraplegia in 1946:

> The paraplegic during the days following his injury is numbed by what has happened to him. One moment he is a healthy, keen, strictly disciplined young man. The next he is gone from the waist down, paralysed, insensitive, unable to fulfil the basic requirements of life in terms of emptying his bladder and bowels. He is fully dependent upon those around him. It is a shattering experience ... Eventually, he arrives in Canada. The journey has been an exhausting one by hospital ship and hospital train. A multitude of problems beset such a patient. Pressure sores commonly developed during the period of evacuation. Practically every patient arriving in Canada had a pressure sore . . . Suprapubic cystotomy had been done on all patients with serious spinal cord injury. Sexual function is abolished and many men are fearful of meeting their fiancées or

wives. This combination of circumstances produces a feeling of lassitude, inertia and despondency.[2]

The horrors of the nature and extent of the injuries even after treatment was a concern: the damage was permanent and traumatizing, even after patients went through several hospitals for treatment. The hospital trains gave the earliest interventions, but the loss had already occurred. For people in Europe, the hospital trains were the first on the scene, but in North America, they were the last, as the *Repository* reminded modern readers on July 28, 2009:

> "After triage on the front lines, depending on where they were, they may have gone to a field hospital, then a hospital ship, which took two weeks, and then they arrived at ports up and down the East Coast from Halifax to Charleston, S.C.," said Framingham's historian, Fred Wallace.
>
> Hospital trains took the wounded for the final leg of their trip.
>
> "There was a railroad spur that crossed Fountain Street that came up directly onto the hospital grounds," Wallace said.
>
> While patients suffered from lost limbs, burns and brain and spinal cord injuries, the town of Framingham reached out to them.[3]

Medical staff on the trains focused on caring for the wounded in the gentlest way possible—and, as reported in Australia's *Hillston Spectator and Lachlan River Advertiser* on August 16, 1945, that constant reassurance was offered even after the war was over: "Red Cross Representative Rogers hands out comforts and amenities to patients returning to their home state by hospital train. Red Cross gives services on all hospital trains."[4]

Newspaper reports emphasized the efficiency of transport, describing the volume of patients and the speed and frequency of the regular trips to the larger medical centres to rescue and salvage the populace. It was an important reassurance, whether the trains were in the middle of a war or in the centre of peace. The egalitarian rescue was the bottom line that mattered; articles as such one in the *Sausalito News* on May 17, 1945, provide an example of how the public's concerns were allayed:

> The Ninth Service Command hospital train unit in one month made 113 trips and moved 1,531 soldier patients a total of 420,405 miles, it was announced today at headquarters, Fort Douglas, Utah.[5]

The hospital trains were a miniature and mobile version of a traditional hospital, and despite being a compact medical centre, it performed the same functions, though sometimes there were trains where a medical student would be the de facto physician making life and death decisions. These mobile units could perform the same multiple functions, from operations to resetting broken bones; they could even be makeshift maternity wards or crude rehabilitation clinics if necessary. The staff on these trains were intervenors and advocates for those who were the most vulnerable and closest to death.

But despite the urgent mandate, hospital trains also symbolized levity and optimism, just as they did the in Great War. No one resented their presence as it meant that there was still a chance of survival, even when there was a catastrophe. As the *Globe and Mail* reported on August 4, 1941, the trains were omens of better things to come:

> The first hospital train to enter Toronto in this war steamed into Union Station last night, bringing back to familiar scenes some of the men who left the city a year ago and more for the battlefront of Europe.
>
> Eighty-five veterans clambered down from the C.N.R. special which had brought them from an East Coast Canadian port. Four others were gently removed on stretchers and placed in ambulances which took them to military hospital.
>
> Back to a peaceful, comfortable city, ablaze with lights, the streets filled with cars, came these

Canadian soldiers, the memory of other cities and other sounds still vivid in their minds. They were tired and grimy from the long journey which saw their ten-car train given right-of-way over all traffic.[6]

The vivid piece made no attempt to hide the extent of trauma, but it also conveyed the joy the trains delivered to those same soldiers:

The veterans brought with them a breath of war. It was not hard to see that these men had come through a lot of hell in the islands across the sea. Some had been blitzed. Some were wounded by shrapnel. Here was a youth with an empty sleeve. Over there was another, grey-haired at the temples. A shell shock case. But there was nothing sad about these veterans . . . They roared three cheers as the train pulled slowly into the station.[7]

Despite the chaos on the battlefields, there was order. There was a method in the madness that determined which of the broken were taken, when, and where. The most perilously injured were taken first, but there were other lines too. As mentioned previously, the "walking wounded" were collected and rode on their own trains, separated from other kinds of wounded and sick. The *Globe and Mail* described these on March 27, 1944:

There is an atmosphere about hospital trains carrying "walking wounded" that gives them a far less tragic tone than the Red Cross-marked trains transporting stretcher cases from the battlefields of Italy.

Walking wounded is a loose term for men who have seen action but whose injuries have ... left them with an empty sleeve, a missing leg or blinded eyes.[8]

Yet, not everyone who was cared for on the trains made it home alive. Newspaper accounts of the era would give details, including if the soldier died on a train, as the *Fisherman* noted in a February 6, 1945, article about a local British Columbia fisherman and solider who could not hold on long enough:

Badly wounded in France on October 9, Private George Hamilton of Port Alberni, a member of the United Fishermen's Union, died aboard the hospital train that was bringing him to Vancouver.

He passed away just before reaching Winnipeg and was buried with full military honours in that city.[9]

The process of collecting the fallen was a dangerous and never-ending affair. Vicious battles meant increased danger for those on the trains, and yet the hospital trains were often the first responders on the scene. Often, it would be too perilous to respond, leaving the most injured close to death. As Feasby recounted in 1956:

> The many Canadian and British wounded who had so unfortunately to be left at Dieppe were evacuated in the same manner as German casualties. Over an hour before the action finally ended, 150 Canadians and British had been cleared from the battlefield to a field dressing station, along with 130 Germans. Nearly 350 of our wounded were evacuated with some 175 Germans by the first hospital train, which left the Dieppe area early in the evening of 19 August. A second train, dispatched about midnight, carried another 240 Canadians and British. Both trains were well staffed by German medical personnel. During the morning of 20 August, the field dressing station serving the Dieppe area was finally cleared of all but seven German and 16 Canadian casualties, who were so seriously wounded that they could not be moved.[10]

The hospital trains were the first part of the journey to saving the broken and decimated: it was the preface for thousands of soldiers and civilians that gave a hint of what the long road of recovery would entail. The trains were transient and fleeting but bought seconds until a sea, plane or traditional hospital could be reached. The wounded and sick were, in many ways, placed on a medical assembly line, yet despite the depersonalization of the process, the trains got soldiers home. In many cases, the trains represented a circular journey: the broken were rescued by means of hospital trains on the battleground, and when it was time to go back home, it was often a hospital train that ended the journey. It was like a spiral staircase, the journey seemingly repetitive, only those climbing and crawling out ending up in a place higher than where they began.

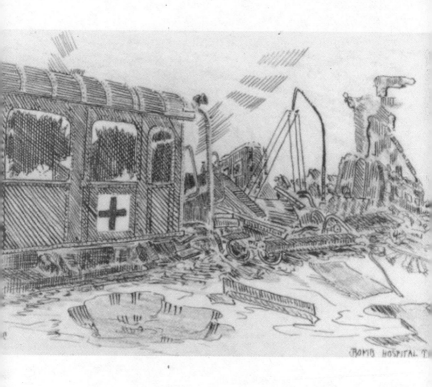

▲ Pencil drawing by James E. Neace depicting the damage to a hospital train after the bombing of Gare Saint-Lazare, Paris, on December 26, 1944. COURTESY OF DAVID NEACE

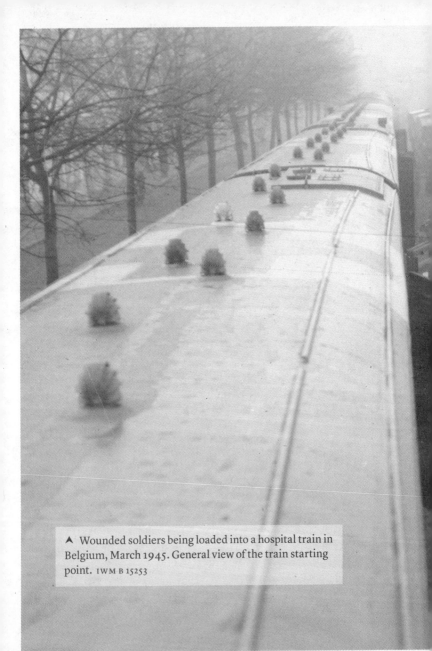

▲ Wounded soldiers being loaded into a hospital train in Belgium, March 1945. General view of the train starting point. IWM B 15253

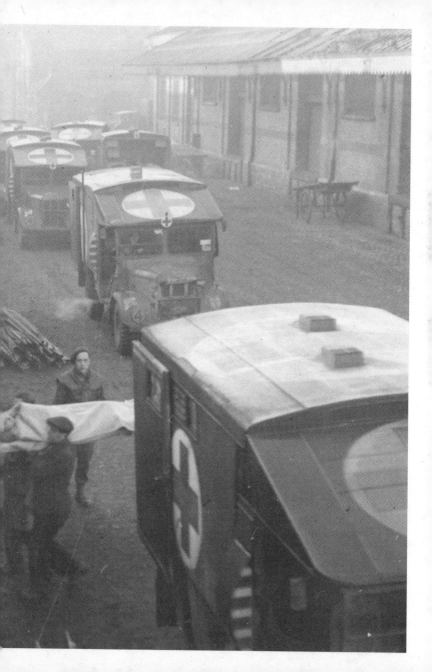

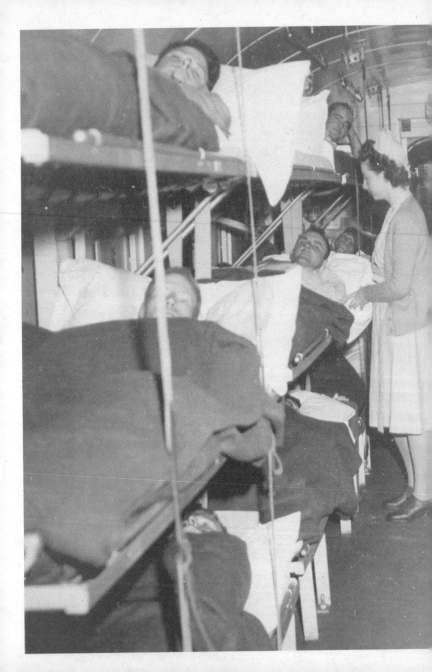

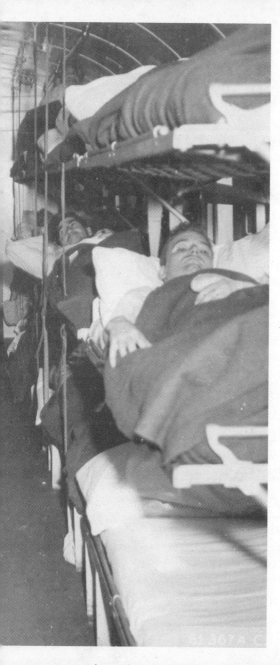

◄ Interior view of a
hospital train showing
wounded Americans.
This picture was taken
after the fall of Brest,
France, on September 4,
1944. US NATIONAL
ARCHIVES, NAID: 204894500

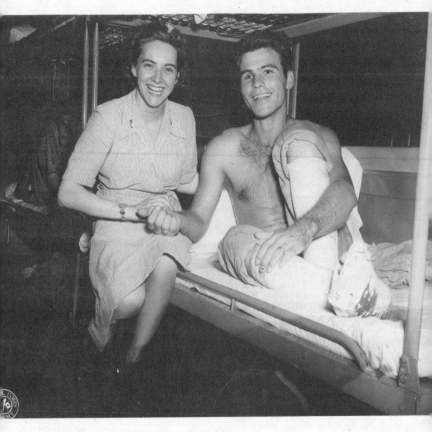

▲ Cpl. James W. Pauley of Sulphur, Oklahoma, is shown in a hospital car with nurse Lt. Bernice Kulp. He was wounded in Italy when he stepped on an anti-personnel mine, fracturing bones in his right foot and left leg and destroying his sight in his right eye. Official photograph US Army Signal Corps, Hampton Roads Port of Embarkation, Newport News, Virginia.

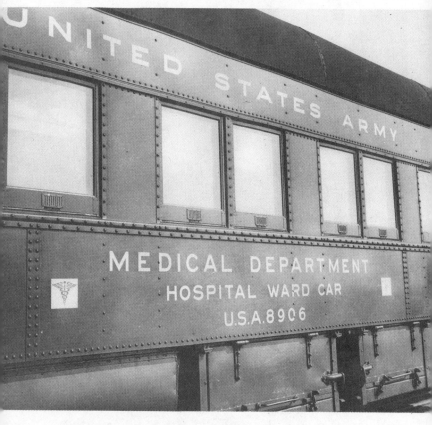

▲ A hospital ward car waiting to be loaded with American wounded returning on transport from Tunisia. Official Photograph US Army Signal Corps, Hampton Roads Port of Embarkation, Newport News Virginia.

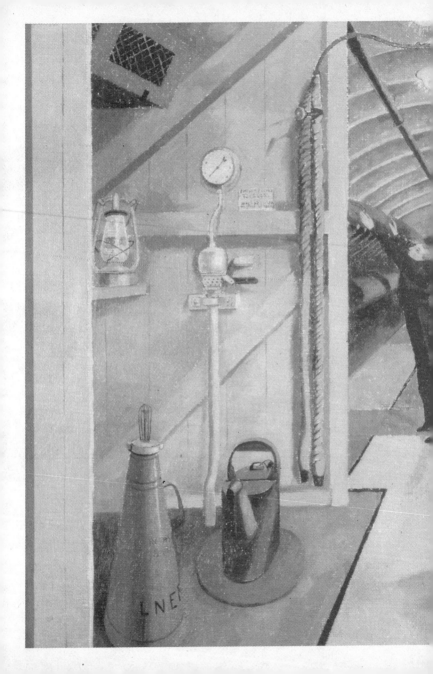

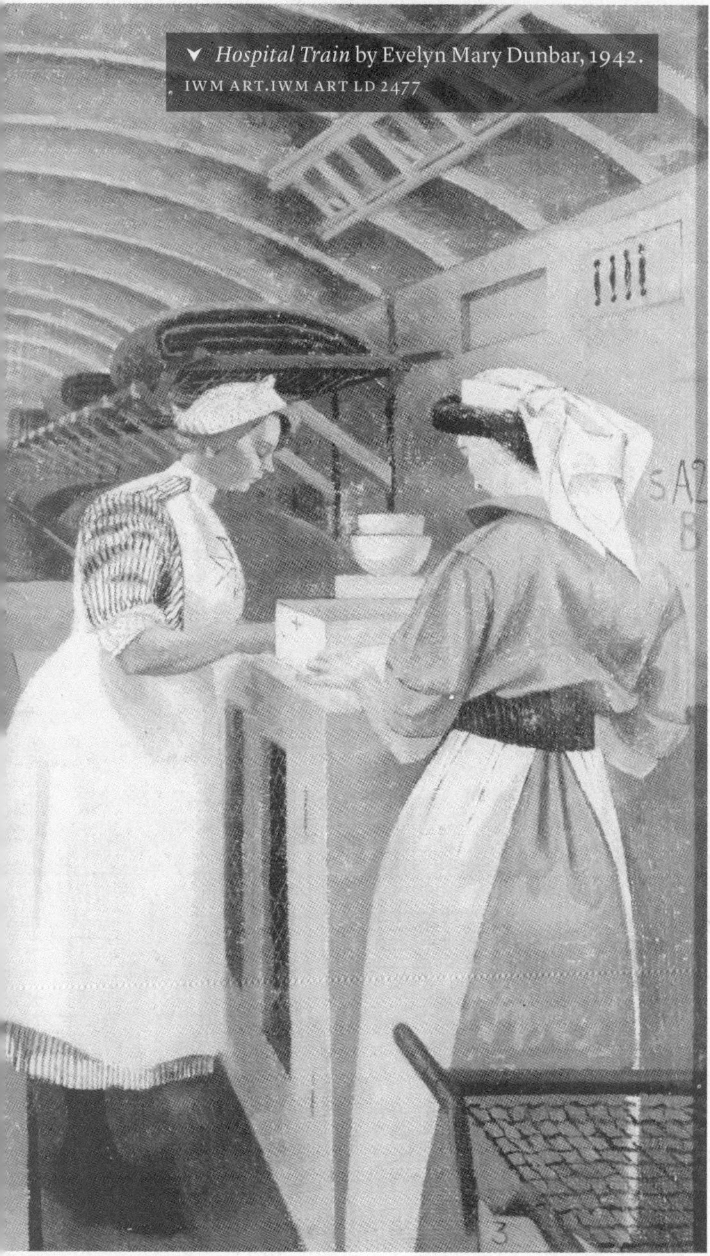

▼ *Hospital Train* by Evelyn Mary Dunbar, 1942.
IWM ART.IWM ART LD 2477

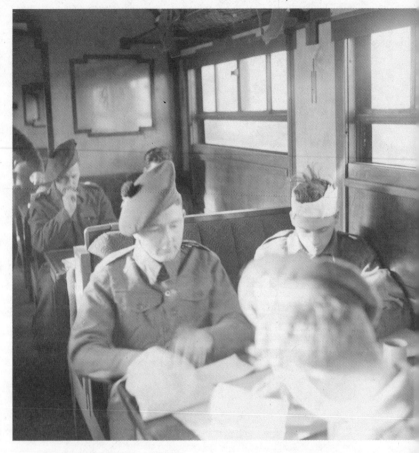

▲ Lightly wounded soldiers playing cards in a hospital train in Belgium. Casualties who were able to walk were given comfortable saloon coaches for the journey. IWM B 15255

➤ Four hospital train nurses of various nationalities enjoying a day off at the Adriatic Coast. The author's grandmother, Stanka Ugrenović, is on the right. COURTESY OF DUSHICA PUHARIC

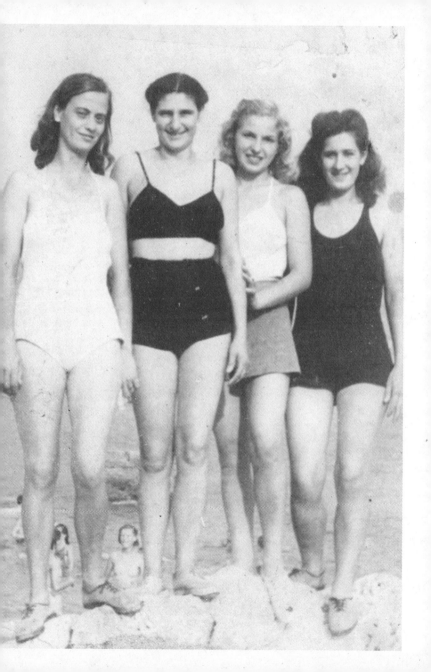

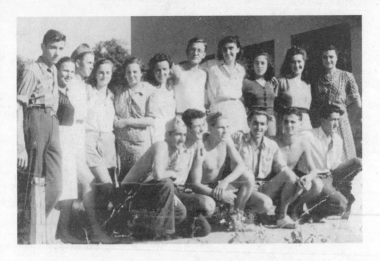

∧ Partisans from the Czech Republic helped hospital train nurses in their mission. The author's grandmother, Stanka Ugrenović, is in the top row, second to the right. COURTESY OF DUSHICA PUHARIC

∨ Several hospital train nurses who took a train of orphans to the Adriatic Coast. The author's grandmother, Stanka Ugrenović, is in the top row, second to the right. COURTESY OF DUSHICA PUHARIC

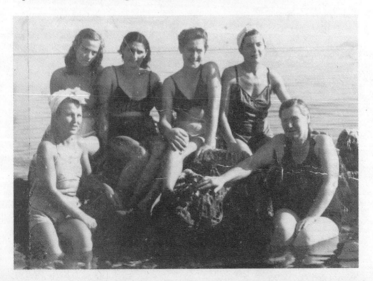

[8]

THE BATTLES

HOSPITAL TRAINS WEAVED IN AND out of conflicts multiple times a day. While most of the time warring factions agreed not to hit the trains, sometimes that promise was broken. One of the most well-known of these acts was on December 26, 1944, when German bombs hit Hospital Train #23 at the Gare Saint-Lazare in Paris, putting the railway station out of service for forty-eight hours. Few artists had dealt with this subject matter, but US medic and colour pencil artist James E. Neace immortalized such a scene in one of his works.

Hospital trains had been the target of other attacks throughout the war. In 1941 alone, for instance, Nazis carried out no fewer than 224 attacks on these trains.[1] Personnel could rarely defend themselves, though sometimes they carried rifles and could fire back. Other times, there was an ambush or danger that came from bombs above. Such a case was reported in the *Wilmington Morning Star* on January 1, 1940:

> Russian air raiders elsewhere spread new death and terror. Red machine gunners splattered a hospital train with lead, the Finns announced officially, and fired on a "clearly marked Red Cross ambulance" from the air.[2]

News of the attack made the front page of the *New York Times* on January 1, 1940, and sent global shockwaves:

> According to private reports, they bombed and machine-gunned the Lutheran Church, but whether or not they killed anybody is not known here tonight ...
> Tonight's communique also said that the Russians made air and artillery attacks on two coastal forts and inflicted slight damage ... there also one was killed and several wounded. The communique also asserts that a hospital train, clearly marked with red crosses, was bombed today.[3]

By their very nature, position, and mandates, hospital trains collided with various battles, and yet they made their way through deadly tribulations as a norm rather than an exception. Railways were sabotaged often during the war, from Poland to Greece to Denmark. Trains were clearly marked with a large red cross, and their schedules were well known to all on the battlefield. But despite sabotage, bombs, infection, disease, lice, rats, and even patient violence making the rides perilous, thousands of lives were still saved throughout the conflict.

Because of the trains' inherent vulnerability to attack, manufacturers had to find ways to maximize the efficiency of all aspects of their construction. Early in the war, there was discourse over size and functionality. A 1940 US *Army Medical Report* editorial debated which design aspect was the most pragmatic:

> Hospital trains are evidently the subject of extensive plans, and a unit has been designed in conjunction with the Pullman Co. for 500 patients. "Such hospital trains will be used ... in the theatre of operations if suitable railway equipment is available." The size of this train is, of course, very convenient if it can be used, but we fear that there may be difficulties in finding sidings available when there is great congestion, as in active operations. There is much to be said for smaller trains and more of them.[4]

Overall, the trains were a success, and the sheer volume of patients moved attested to their ultimate triumph. By the end of the war, a routine was established, and as more battles brought Allied forces closer to victory, the hospital trains functioned more efficiently, despite mechanical problems and dodgy supplies. Those doctors involved with the trains had reverence for the outcome, as Charles M. Walson expressed in the April 1947 issue of *The Military Surgeon*:

> In November 1942 we received two hospital trains. Later additional trains were provided, all of which proved very successful in our evacuation problems. Our Hospital Trains reached their maximum activity during the month of May 1945 when 18,794 patients were carried on 76 trains. Rail shipments were made throughout the US. In two instances we received patients from shipside at Halifax, Nova Scotia. During the last week in May 1945, 37 trains were dispatched, the cars traveling a total of 460,828 miles, which represented 13,824,837, passenger miles.[5]

The results were the confirmation—or refutation—of the theories and endless calculations. The battleground was a laboratory, meaning empirical answers came with each journey on the tracks. How many were recused? How many lived? How many died? Runs were refined, and alterations would be made to the strategies of patient treatment and transport. As author and historian Michael Foley explains, the logistics were precise:

The movement of men and equipment towards the south coast continued after D-Day as the men in Europe still had to be supplied. There was also, however, a large amount of movement in the opposite direction, with hospital trains carrying the wounded back from the south. Many of these were American servicemen. Those who were to be repatriated to America were taken to Liverpool or Glasgow.

There were three hospital trains on constant standby: two American and one British. When ships carrying wounded arrived from France, the hospital trains would be moved to the town quay to load the wounded.[6]

Finding refuge amid conflict was nearly impossible for the healthy, and the sick and wounded were even more vulnerable to death—or capture, often a fate worse than death. The trains' medical personnel didn't hold guns but carried medicine and offered the best option to those in need; after all, to be taken on the train meant safe passage and a chance to heal. As author Cynthia Toman recounts, nurses ensured the most vulnerable were removed from the world's most dangerous conflicts:

As the senior medical and nursing service, it was the army—and not navy nurses—who staffed the Canadian hospital ships (the *Lady Nelson* and *Letitia*) and sick-bay quarters of the *Queen Elizabeth* and *Queen Mary*, transporting soldiers, prisoners of war, and war brides, and thus exacerbating rivalries between the nursing services. Some RCAMC nurses also participated in patient evacuations from the continent to England after D-Day on Dakota and Sparrow airplanes. Others staffed military hospital trains within Canada. Attached to regular passenger trains, hospital trains had specially designed and furnished cars accommodating sixteen to twenty-eight bed patients in addition to "sitting" patients.[7]

Looking after the wounded in the middle of a war is delicate enough, but the constant route by track to the sea could be a treacherous affair. If not a bomb from outside, then an outbreak from within could strike an entire train down. Thankfully, there were safe havens in which to sit back and regroup. While doctors and nurses worried about saving the wounded, generals and governments worried about the logistics to ensure safe passage— and much of the success of the trains rested on fiat and goodwill.

Though there was a tacit understanding that trains with a Red Cross symbol were not to be harmed, the rules would be broken frequently. For example, the June 10, 1940, edition of the *West Australian* reported:

"The wreckage of a hospital train bombed by German airmen in France. Some of the carriages were completely demolished."[8]

The tracks often were more like a roulette wheel than a mode of transportation. Because of the dangers, the trains were seen as an internationally coordinated affair. It was imperative for channels to be open and concessions to be made for the greater good. Those overseeing the operations of the trains could focus on different players and take an active role in determining the level of cooperation, investment, and contribution to its maintenance and service, meaning that success was the norm for the trains:

> By arrangement, the hospital was always able to transfer cases, either by ambulance, convoy or hospital train, to various E.M.S. hospitals, such as Mount Vernon, Stoke Mandeville, Park Prewett, Horton, or even further afield. This was essential in order to keep a number of beds always available for fresh casualties. Cases requiring specialised treatment, such as brain injuries, plastic surgery or chest surgery could always be transferred to the special units for these cases at E.M.S. Hospitals, Mount Vernon, Horton and East Grinstead. On one occasion, a case of suppurative pericarditis was dealt with by a mobile chest unit operating team from Epsom.[9]

But not all was peaceful or cooperative among the Allies: France charged a steep toll for the use of their tracks, including hospital trains that were often already low on supplies and required speed to get through. In general, the trains were an expensive enterprise—and one whose success was not marked financially, but by the number of lives saved.

Keeping trains clean was nearly unattainable, despite the lavish praise from the press. Yet unsanitary conditions were just one of many dangers that personnel had to battle—personnel who were young, inexperienced, and often had never left home prior to the war. As author Nicola Tyrer describes, the trains had to face battles that came from everywhere, without respite:

> For much of the war, waged from the air or from under the sea as much as on land, there was no front line—the enemy attacked indiscriminately. Between 1939 and 1945, wherever there were Allied troops risking their lives, there were QAs. A thousand newly enlisted qas went over with the British Expeditionary Force in 1939. Trapped in the lightning advance of the Germans as they invaded Holland and Belgium, they rescued thousands of wounded British troops by loading them onto hospital trains—trains that might later be blown up or bombed. At the docks they helped carry the injured

onto waiting hospital ships under wave after wave of attacks by the Luftwaffe.[10]

The UK's Royal Naval Medical Service noted in 1954 that medical strategy was required, assuring increased chances of survival, regardless of gunfire or air raids:

> To convey the patients from the airfields to the C.C.S. a pool of twenty-five ambulances was set up at Yatesbury and a wireless transmission channel was maintained between Yatesbury and Wroughton, as it was considered that this would be the most efficient and expeditious method of controlling the ambulances. In practice, however, the W.T. channel was found to be redundant and it was eventually closed down. Teams of stretcher-bearers were provided to off-load casualties at the C.C.S. and to on-load them again when convoys had been made up for transfer by road or by hospital train from Shrivenham siding. Initially, twenty-five aircrew pupils from a nearby training centre were utilised but at a later date fifty Italian co-operators were employed and this arrangement was found to be satisfactory. Considerable care was devoted to the training of these personnel, as the efficient working of the C.C.S. depended greatly upon the rapid and careful unloading of the casualties.[11]

In North Africa in 1942, trains were an important lifeline, as recounted in 1961 by Leonard D. Heaton, then Surgeon General for the US Army, in his annual report:

The 1st Battalion of the 16th Medical Regiment, with the assistance after 18 February of the British 6th Motor Ambulance Convoy, operated an ambulance shuttle from Tébessa to Constantine, approximately 140 miles. The same road served as a main supply route for II Corps. Beginning in mid-March, the 16th Medical Regiment also staffed and operated a French hospital train, which ran from Tébessa to Ouled Rahmoun, just south of Constantine, where the narrow-gauge Tébessa line intercepted the main east–west railroad. A traffic control post at Aïn Mlilla distributed patients from ambulance convoys and hospital trains to vacant beds in the area. In the northern sector the ambulance route of the 16th Medical Regiment ran eighty-five miles from Tabarka to Bône. Rail evacuation from the northern sector was by two British hospital trains from Souk el Khemis, each with capacity for 120 litter and 200 sitting patients.[12]

Each successful mission added to the confidence of the mobile units, regardless of where they rode and how many they carried to safety. Yet the spectacle and symbolism of the trains could be used for more pragmatic purposes in an effort to rally troops or boost morale. They could become shorthand for whatever narrative someone wished. Journalists often could take advantage of the icon to shade their work:

> The following day, [CBS reporter William] Shirer claimed to have observed another long Red Cross train unloading wounded and received word of two more at Charlottenburg. This contemporary account, by a highly reputable journalist, is not easily dismissed, although precisely what Shirer witnessed first-hand beyond "several airmen" remains ambiguous. Shirer later concluded the men in Berlin were casualties of an exercise surprised by the RAF but it should be borne in mind that he was actively pro-British, and was thanked by name in the official history of BSC in New York, written in 1945. The suspicion therefore remains that in 1941 Shirer deliberately exaggerated the hospital train story as a morale booster, at a time when the war was going particularly badly for Britain. Curiously, there exist apparently reliable reports of similar trains seen at the Gare du Nord in Brussels at about the same time. Yet even the most hardened conspiracy theorist must baulk [sic] at the notion that, in the years since 1945, all mention of a

large-scale amphibious disaster to rival the Dieppe raid in 1942 can have been expunged from every memoir, unit history and official file.[13]

The battles fought among soldiers were only one set of clashes hospital trains had to contend with, yet these would require transparency and diplomacy. Being so open with plans was risky, yet it was a reason for the trains' success. Cooperation and coordination from the train to those outside it were critical:

Twenty hospital trains arrived at Kidderminster in 1944. The camp had been there before the war and was once visited by General Patton. The wounded men were unloaded in the sidings at Kidderminster under armed guard. Locals knew when a train was on its way as all the points were clamped to allow access.[14]

As well, the key to the success of the hospital trains was the US's dedication to ensuring physical cars were brought in. This mission did not go unnoticed or unappreciated. As Brigadier J.G. Morgan noted in *Notes from a War Diary: The Isle of Wight and Tripoli* in 1942:

Although the hospital trains were pulled by LNER locomotives, the Americans had also brought their own locomotives with them as they began to build up their supplies for D-Day. Most of the American engines had been used to pull goods trains. They were painted grey and either had Transportation Corps USA or just USA painted on them. Although many of them had gone to France, some American engines remained in England.[15]

While weapons of combat required planning, so too did the flow and operations of the trains. Even if supplies were low and disease was a threat, the operations had to be optimized from every angle under control. Brigadier Morgan had to make careful calculations of where the trains went to ensure a successful outcome:

I had taken over the Ryde Pier Hotel as a hospital and staffed it with BRC and St Johns volunteers. I made an ambulance train to take the overflow from there to Totland Bay. I went to the Royal Yacht Squadron and arranged with them for a boat to evacuate casualties to the mainland. My initial appraisal had concluded that any raid was most likely to take place on Cowes where two new destroyers were under construction and I therefore planned the evacuation routes on this basis. I also made the Prison into a CCS Operating Theatre.[16]

Despite his best efforts, limitations were plentiful and difficult to overcome, frustrating him:

> With the lines of communication so stretched, a severe strain was placed on arrangements for evacuation of wounded, but I was dismayed to find that the hospital trains from Alexandria were dirty. I generally tidied up hygiene and administration. I saw the need for some method of recording wounded and deciding which beds they were to go to and seeing that one hospital was not overloaded whilst another was under-deployed.[17]

Yet despite many battles and victories, history still keeps its secrets. We know very little of the experience of certain sociocultural and ethnic groups among the different military forces. For example, on July 1, 1944, the *Mississippi Enterprise* briefly reported:

> The following [Black] patients were among the sixteen oversea veterans who arrived Tuesday afternoon on a hospital train from Hareran General Hospital, Los Angeles for recuperation in Foster General Hospital: Pvt. Henry C. May, Laurel; Pfc. T. C. Walker, West Point; Pfc. James K. Dillard, Vicksburg.[18]

Unfortunately, very little remains of such records, and as such, historians are denied a wealth of information.

The peculiar symbiotic relationship between the hospital trains and the battleground merged the best and the worst of humanity. While warring factions fought one another, those on the trains fought death and despair. Those who worked on the trains had the biggest stakes of them all, and while the hospital trains lost many a battle, in the end, they won the war. People lived, and in the end, that was the only thing that mattered.

[9]

THE FUTURE IS PAST

WHAT IS CONSIDERED ARCHAIC BY one generation was once cutting edge to the generation of the past. Jet engines took off as a force during the Second World War. The use of radar and electronic computers also began there. The Jeep, the microwave oven, and even the atomic bomb had their debut and traction in this era. While these are all now woven into the mundane global fabric, once upon a time, these were shocking forays into an unknown future. These contraptions were seen as tools for good if in the right hands, but should there be defeat by an enemy, they could also be used for evil. Ambiguity built suspense as much as it could build hope and confidence.

Hospital trains were nestled between the realm of the mundane familiar and the futuristic innovative. While mobile hospitals had been in use prior to the Second World War, they were presented as a true engineering breakthrough and were interpreted as a sign of techno-logical advancement. Interestingly enough, the hybrid narrative of the trains would gain public trust, but also goodwill and faith at once. There was enough com-fort for the jittery risk-aversive to believe in the power of the trains, but also enough for the more daring to embrace the trains' status as future-oriented.

The construction of the trains was fluid, and plans could quickly be modified or scuttled if something better came along, as the United States Army, European Theater of Operations unit noted in 1945:

> The first American hospital train to sup-port the invasion was improvised from the French 40-and-8s. These cars were discarded when Cherbourg was opened and the modern trains arrived from England. Typical of the 47 trains built by the French and British for the US Army Medical Department was "Old 27," staffed by Hospital Train Group No. 43. This outfit brought the first hospital train to the Continent, was first into Paris and Belgium with it, blazed the way into Germany.[1]

The trains could be used to sort patients, creating a myth of specialization to the public in subtextual ways:

Back on the beaches and hards of England, casualties were sorted and immediately dispatched to installations prepared to administer the type of medical attention required. Patients whose condition permitted were loaded into ambulances and driven to transit hospitals. More seriously wounded were moved to hospitals set up near the port. There, patients were treated for shock, X-rayed, operated [on].[2]

Finally, simple coordination allowed for a workflow which suggested that organization in chaos added to the notions of superior analytical thinking, stemming from the union of science, medicine, and engineering over brute strength:

Patients remained at these installations until they could make the journey inland to general hospitals where definitive treatment could be administered. The overall procedure was coordinated with train schedules and space available in the hospitals.[3]

The advantage of movement, volume, and positive outcomes had a positive effect on the image of the hospital train. Despite being tethered to a track, the concept proved to be effective in lowering the number by dead, hence removing some of the terror in the bargain. Death was not a foregone conclusion. But how did hospital trains become a symbol of the future of technology?

Some inspiration came from a desire to tweak the nose of the enemy—essentially, the German regime looked down on the trains, so the Allies saw more value in having them. Many elites before the war didn't believe trains had value and, hence, dismissed them, giving an advantage to those who saw an opportunity. In his 1956 article in *Military Medicine*, Oscar P. Dost explains how Germany had seen the railways as obsolete:

> Between 1930–1940, in wide circles of the trans-portation administrators, the view was held that the railroad had become strategically obsolete and that, especially in the field of transportation of the sick, it could be equally or more advantageously replaced by automobiles. These circles were taught differ-ently in a rather drastic way, however, since their refusal in preparing a sufficient number of all types of hospital trains resulted in the loss of many lives.[4]

Those who saw the value of trains were ignored and even censored, but it did not stop others from making use of the same sage advice:

> We German railway specialists had repeatedly attempted to persuade our national socialistic

government on the urgent need to prepare and to set up a sufficient number of hospital trains. Shortly before World War II and in the first years of that war, I published five essays on this subject, but further articles were not permitted to appear. Yet, those published may have had some effect, and may have helped some people in the world.[5]

The trains had one more strategic advantage in that they could bring people together in that future-forward vision, associating hospital trains with a bright future rather than a grim dystopian one:

Here there was Englishmen against Englishmen, Germans against Germans, brother against brother; they had battled with fanaticism and not always in a fair manner. BUT—and this is absolutely unique in the entire military history of the world—there occasionally shone a beam of light of human dignity and love of neighbor; ways and means were found to make hospital trains available for both the combat lines. The hospital train, under the observance of certain recognizable marks and rules, e.g., a red and white lamp, was considered neutral; it moved between the combat lines to pick up the wounded. Where else had anything like this occurred? Where else had so much humanity been exhibited in war?

While many things seem to have been forgotten, the transportation of the sick and wounded has been recognized as due to the Americans.[6]

The US's rise as a global avatar of innovation and competence has much to do with the triumphs in all sectors of the Second World War. From the weapons of mass destruction to the tools of healing, it seemed that the US had a near monopoly on setting the new terms of the debate on the trains' usefulness. This scaffolding of power and influence can be seen in the modern era, and the US involvement in the manufacture and use of the trains in Europe left a distinct impression on the global collective psyche. While few things about the trains remain in memory, the origin of the trains' creation remains firmly in place.

Yet, how did the trains help shape the US's reputation during the conflict? For one, the sheer volume of patients that could be handled at any given time made it seem that hospitals could become portable while retaining the ability to administer the latest medication and procedures. Casualties could be quickly brought into the trains which were always on the move and close to the fighting.

Second, hospital trains employed the latest medicines or procedures of the time to treat the most injured. The trains were not an inferior version of the traditional hospital, meaning the best possible care would be provided until the patients could reach a larger centre. And, as schedules and efficiency ensured the best chances of survival, soldiers were, perhaps subconsciously, more willing to take bigger risks. As John Hedley-Whyte and Debra R. Milamed explain in their 2014 article in the *Ulster Medical Journal*, there was a greater plan in place:

> The plans for evacuation of wounded and sick led to delineation of Army and Navy responsibility in LSTs, other Allied vessels and on the beaches and harbours on both sides of the Channel and the Irish Sea. The roles and availability of motors, aircraft and Hospital Trains were discussed and priorities assigned. The transfer of wounded to RAMC, US Army, US Navy and Royal Navy Hospitals was planned. In general, the Navies would be responsible for their own wounded and the Armies for both soldiers and airmen and wounded Prisoners of War. Standards for potable water and milk, their testing and procurements in Normandy, were enacted. Plans for treatment of tuberculosis and gas gangrene and the deployment of penicillin and sulfonamides and above all blood and plasma were delineated. "Whole blood will be an item of medical supply and will be distributed through medical supply channels. It will be given the highest priority in transportation." A

ten-day supply of blank forms and stationery were to be stocked in advance dumps and a month's supply in Base Depots.[7]

The US was at the forefront of these units, and its consistent superiority in battle wins, strategies, and tools was noticed by everyone. The UK, too, had managed to show its abilities when it came to the hospital trains. The trains built the credibility of those who had jockeyed for prominence in a postwar era and showed foresight and a vision of the future.

But in the end, it was the sturdiness of the trains which gave the most hope and confidence to both soldiers and civilians. There was a sense of trust in everything from the materials that made the train to the abilities of the people who worked inside them. Joseph R. Darnall, recounting events from October 1944 four years later in the October 1948 edition of *Military Surgeon*, explains that nothing was certain around him save for the train:

In the heart of the city, near the river and railway station, we paused to inquire of an M.P. the direction to the 15th General Hospital. While talking to the M.P., there was a terrific explosion which jarred our vehicle and bounced the M.P.'s motorcycle off the concrete.

The explosion was followed immediately by an intense tremulous swishing sound, characteristic of the new V-2 rocket bombs. The missile had struck not far from the railway station where two hospital trains were being loaded. No patients or crew members were hurt by the blast, but many expressed eagerness to accelerate their departure for Paris.[8]

Considering the damage and destruction, it was only the trains that could haul many people to safety at once:

A terrific load was being thrust upon the 15th General Hospital. It was accepting all patients requiring hospitalization, and the staff had been working under tremendous pressure for ten days and nights. More than a thousand battle casualties were hauled in by ambulance and admitted in one day, while another thousand were evacuated from this installation to hospital trains and ambulance planes for shipment to Paris. For days and weeks, the 15th General was obliged to function as an extremely busy evacuation hospital.[9]

In many ways, the trains were the vanguard of egalitarian medical care: doctors made house calls, and it was entirely feasible for the hospital to do so, too. The trains saved lives and changed the fortunes of both individuals and nations; however, the message was a quiet one, without the usual bombast messaging of the era. There were no "hospital train heroes" presented in the press. There was no overt spokesperson who spoke to the press. The trains did not have nicknames or extraordinary claims to fame. The abilities of the train and those who worked in them was assumed. Everything was taken for granted, and the quiet heroics of those who worked on the trains hinted that after their use was maximized and peace returned, the trains would all but vanish from public consciousness.

10

THE SECRET SOCIAL

DESPITE THE DANGER WROUGHT BY war, within and
without—and because of it—hospital trains were more
than mere assembly lines or "chop shops." Personal
bonds were forged, and the trains became a sanctuary for
the kind-hearted, whose own reality seemed to turn cru-
elly against them. The point of the trains was to save lives
and preserve morale, and it took emotionality to ensure
that mandate could be fulfilled. Many gravitated to the
gentlest people for companionship and support; the care
given involved not only physical rescue but also showing
those who had lost limbs that they had as much inherent
value as when their bodies were whole. Emotional currency was as important as primal currency.

The hospital trains were settings of life and death, but
there could be a certain jovial air about them. Pecking
orders took a backseat as reality proved that titles meant

little when there was carnage; what mattered was a good nature and connection. As scholar Jane Brooks explains in her 2019 essay in the book *Negotiating Nursing*, even in the postscript of the Second World War, those who had humility and purpose could thrive emotionally:

> Anxieties about the end of the war resound through many of the nurses' testimonies. Sister Catherine Butland reflected on it being "regretful that the seven months just past could not go in indefinitely, though very glad the fighting was over." However, for many nurses the war did not end in 1945, but as late as 1947. In the latter months and immediate post-war period, the needs of POWs, civilian inmates in concentration camps and the millions of starving people across the globe were to concentrate the minds and skills of some nursing sisters and provide further valuable work. In August 1946, Sister Ann Radloff was posted to a hospital train in Palestine. As she had been in the Army for over two years, she was designated "Officer Commanding Train." Although she admits that she had never "felt less in command of anything" and that "no one took me seriously," her position, even nominally being in charge of anything but a hospital ward contravened normal professional and gender rules and would have made Radloff's return to

pre-war hierarchies challenging. She was demobilised in 1947 after "three years of exciting, terrifying and varying experiences. I look back in gratitude for the friendship and camaraderie of which I was part."[1]

Having a good nature went a long way on the ride and allowed people to bond under the worst of circumstances. The trains became a hub to bond and build camaraderie, and their importance in reinforcing social bonds cannot be ignored. There was a sense of adventure and common purpose that transcended job roles. Cooks and porters on the trains, as well as medical personnel, were often young people, some still in their teens, and together they shared a sense of adventure, despite the danger—or precisely because of it. Eros and Thanatos are somehow linked in our brains on a primal level; when there is death, there is life and love to be taken at every and any given chance as it may never come again.

Even in the darkest of rides, there was innocence, even playfulness. These wild and young adventurers and altruists were determined to make a difference while finding meaning in the rubble. As one woman recounted in 2016, the way of the trains defined her late grandmother:

My grandfather is no longer alive, but I know his story from my grandmother, Lyudmila Azhnina. She left for the front as a volunteer when she was

17, having lied about her age. Her surname was still Smirnova. She was deployed to a hospital train and she had to get used to her fear of the sky: The fascist planes would fly right over the train and bomb it, aiming at the bright red crosses on the wagon roofs.

It is painful for my grandmother to remember whatever is related to death and fear. More often she talks about ordinary stories: how everyone would sing and dance during the stops when there was no shooting; or how she wrote home: "Sell everything, just so there is enough to buy food!"[2]

The trains brought strangers from every continent and nation together, and humility and humour were the glue that held bonds in place. In close quarters, amid uncertainty and danger, laughter could be heard frequently. The youths who worked on the trains refused to bow or to break to the darkness of war; this was why fortunes turned around. As Australian Army nurse Lorna Laffer recalled in 1995, the trains were imperfect, yet incubated a sense of bravery and levity at once:

> No doubt a hospital train conjures up in your minds smooth-running carriages, air-conditioned and silent, chromium-plated appointments, indirect lighting and sliding doors! But let me tell you of our

own special model in the troubled wartime days of 1942 in North Australia.

It was after the bombing of Darwin, and another Sister and I of the Australian Army Nursing Service lived a roving mobile life in "Leaping Lena," the train which had been converted from cattle trucks. Despite the unreliable "iron horses" which drew her gasping and grunting on slippery rails, or careening down inclines at what seemed breakneck speed, we grew fond of this rattling contraption, as it swayed its uncertain way.[3]

Those who worked on the trains and the ones rescued by them had time to talk, eat together, and even sing; they were defined by living with strangers in close quarters, flaws and all. Death and danger never left those who rode the trains, yet their defiance proved effective. The danger was outside of the trains, but also very much within them with the risk of disease outbreaks. Nothing was predictable or easy. But the bonds forged through trauma healed many as they navigated out of the war.

The trains brought a sense of connection to communities who made it their purpose to rally around their operation and existence. Pharmacists in the US made it a goal to "sell $1,000,000 worth of War Bonds to build a hospital train to transport wounded men," according to the *La Jolla Journal* on April 6, 1944.[4] The trains were a source of honour and pride, and in a subsequent article on April 13, the method of fundraising was clearly an appeal to connect to community:

> "Help Buy a Hospital Train" is the caption of a poster now being circulated by the druggists of Southern California, who are sponsoring a move by their association to pay for a fully equipped hospital train, the total cost of which is estimated at one million dollars.
>
> Druggists of the Southland have set their quota at the amount named above, and the local pharmacists are desirous that those buying bonds should purchase one or more at the local stores.
>
> The local quota has been set at $3000.[5]

Fundraisers succeeded as communities held events to join a just cause, making the trains a reason for social cohesion in battle and elsewhere. Those who had previously come home by hospital train often returned to the station to watch others like them return. Many of those working on the trains on battlefields would also go out and socialize among themselves and in the towns where they stopped to gather supplies. Train personnel would befriend farmers and others to ensure more than just supplies and safe passage, but also to keep a sense of community alive amid the stench of death and destruction.

Because the mandate of the hospital trains was to preserve life and cheat death, those who were saved by the trains began to take that mandate into their own essence of being. Humanity fuelled the trains and ensured the ethos of benevolence was continued. The message that healing people would help win the war could be conveyed not by military might, but by good old-fashioned selflessness and altruism. For instance, author Bob Carruthers recounts the journey of one soldier, Leo Mattowitz, who was seriously injured during the Russian winter:

> I was put into a hospital train, together with men who had suffered horrific injuries. Some of them had arms missing. Some of them had trodden on mines and had their feet or their legs blown off. They were unloaded in the field hospitals at Smolensk, Vitebsk and Minsk.
>
> I was in the first wagon behind the engine, and it was hellishly cold; I could walk, but it was so cold that I blacked out … When I'd recovered, I learned that the ones who could walk, like me, were taken to large towns like Brest-Litovsk, Warsaw or Trier … They gave me whatever medicines they had—of course, there was no penicillin at that time—but what they gave me seemed to help.[6]

His recovery was harrowing, but his survival ensured his humanity and connection to others as he paid his gratitude forward:

At another station along the line, some Red Cross nurses brought in food. It wasn't much—half a loaf of army bread, tins of sardines, sausage and pork—but most of the men couldn't eat it. They had bullet wounds in their legs, arms or heads and they were unable to move.

The engine driver said to me, "I have three children at home and there is very little to eat there. Couldn't you give me a bit of bread or get some of the tins of pork for me?" "Yes, I will," I said. I got a backpack, went from section to section and asked, "Are you going to eat that?" "No, you can eat it." When my backpack was full, I took it to the engine driver. He fell around my neck and kissed me and said, "When the trains gets to a big town, come to the engine; I'll hide you and take you all the way to Trier, my home town."[7]

People connected and even stayed together for decades after the trains carried their last patients, with many soldiers trekking to the homes of the nurses and doctors who saved them. Friendships were made, and bonds were cemented. Even for those who never made the journey to reconnect with other patients or medical staff, they understood that they were not alone. The trains transported them to a place outside of death, and they shared a belief that their collective journeys still had many miles to go. Life takes people in many different directions, but for the briefest moment in time, people converged on the trains where those tracks defied the hatred, anger, and fear on the battlegrounds and sped toward a kinder direction. Those who rode them together shared a secret hope and defiance that showed them that, in their hearts, they would never be alone again. There were those who looked for strangers who had strayed too far away for too long, and that was the secret rebellion that defied war and death itself.

11

THE IMAGE

IT WAS NEVER JUST THE nuts and bolts of the trains that gave them the edge and the power to turn global fortunes around, however subtly. It was always about the *aura*. Just as trains were used time and again by fascists for evil intent, it was imperative to counter those frightful connotations with a symbol of health, strength, heroism, and most importantly, triumph. Battles never were just about the soldiers, but also the image of those who were risking their lives to save those soldiers: every symbol was up for grabs, and whichever side won *that* battle was well on the way to winning the war.

Far from being mere moving medical units, the trains were used to boost the morale of the public in the US and Europe. Their symbolism was too powerful to ignore, and in times of rationing and primal survival, nothing could be wasted. Every step mattered. Citizens were under siege, and it was essential that positive messages would give hope to those on the edge of despair.

The role of the press in covering hospital trains cannot be overstated: newspapers on two continents gave citizens vital information and insight into the peculiar world of mobile hospitals during the world's darkest hours, yet the information was presented with optimism. While hospital trains had been in significant use during the First World War, it was not until the Second that they seemed to take on an inspiring persona: the active saviour in modern chaos. The trains were presented as being humbly divine: they were the vehicles that could heal the sick, or at the very least, buy them time until they could reach a stationary hospital or another mobile unit at sea. They were powerful, fast, and inside them were capable and brave men and women who could turn fortunes around in the battlefield at the last possible second. The *Globe and Mail* had quietly chronicled hospital trains in numerous articles, usually with emotionality at its core. A June 26, 1944, headline—"Soldier on Hospital Train Cheered by Fiancée's Welcome"— represents the narrative framing used throughout the war: when the train made a stop, happiness would arrive in the form of love and human connection. The article went on to describe the reunited couple, Corporal Tom Kelly and Miss Nancy Wright, as "blissful and happy" and "wonderful" as Kelly "clutched" Miss Wright the moment he arrived.[1]

The article could have conveyed the same sentiment without revealing how he arrived, yet such powerful symbolism would have been lost. The *Globe and Mail* used the same framing in an earlier piece on April 15, headlined "Throng Cheers Veterans Home from War Zones." The hospital train was transformed into a symbol of happy resolution, regardless the condition of the soldiers being brought home were in:

> Back from the battlefronts, 77 wounded men rolled into Toronto at 1 o'clock in the morning on a hospital train. Thirty-two were stretcher cases.
>
> With a throng cheering them as they marched into the Reception Centre, the walking wounded came on crutches, with patches across an eye or with an empty sleeve.[2]

It was essential to show the might of the trains; however, these news reports emphasized the train without mention of the personnel who looked after the wounded. By the tail end of the war, the doctors and nurses faded from news reports as the trains themselves became a shorthand for them. By this time, the hospital trains themselves became icons and the stars of the narrative: it was all about triumph at the edge of a cataclysm. The trains frequently brought in soldiers without limbs, and yet the news reports emphasized happier times ahead.

The focus on the trains themselves was an unfair shift away from the men and women who ensured soldiers came home in the first place. But this erasure was only the beginning: eventually, the trains too would be lost to the sands of time once Allied victory was assured.

By 1949, the shift in focus was the quiet sign that the trains would slowly be erased from the global public consciousness, and eventually, their value as a symbol of hope would fade away—not because of the trains' failure, but because of their success in reducing the number of dead. While the trains would still make headlines and be in the top position of the journalistic inverted pyramid, everything started to align to a new story arc, one that drifted away from the darkness of war. The trains arrived and delivered, but when they took their final bow, there was no expectation of an encore, nor even the slightest acknowledgement of their existence. The latter tacit collective decision would be the most historically troubling; after all, it was the nurses, the women, who were most closely associated with the power of hospital trains as they were the front-line workers who had the most contact with the wounded and ill. Regardless of their triumph in reducing the number of casualties, their successes would not be leveraged to maintain or expand their personal freedoms. Their immediate postwar future was a regression in freedoms and mobility, and the clearest evidence of their independence would be conspicuously kept out of the public consciousness and history books for decades.

Nevertheless, the singular role of hospital trains as an image of hope during the war was unequivocal. The unspoken heroes who worked on them demonstrated that death was not a foregone conclusion. More intriguingly, the personnel held a quiet but bigger power that wasn't openly recognized but was tacitly acknowledged in the hundreds of news reports during the war. The soldiers who fought on the battlefield had advantages over regular citizens, yet illness and injury became an equalizer where the fortunes of both civilians and soldiers would ultimately be in the hands of healers. In the world of fighting and destruction, the ultimate deal-makers were those who saved lives in hospitals, but in the hierarchy, those in trains were on top of the order. The brick-and-mortar hospitals and hospital ships were inaccessible for millions of people, while the trains were able to come out to look for the fallen when they strayed too far for too long.

The press at the time emphasized the power and resilience of the trains to the point of idolization, yet there were specific themes and focus on the stories, regardless of the media outlet or even nation. Stories focused on both those who manufactured the trains and the nurses who worked on them, both being lauded for their singular abilities. In one November 26, 1943, *Globe and Mail* article headlined "Hospital Train Unique From Safety Standpoint," the focus was on both singularity and practicality:

> Home and family and all else that a fighting man dreams about are nearing reality hour by hour, as this 18-car army hospital train steams slowly westward through the Maritimes.
>
> Among the war-scarred patients are the first group of Canadian prisoners-of-war repatriated from Germany and a number of officers and men who took part in the Sicilian campaign.
>
> Life aboard this train is as comfortable as it is humanly possible to make it. More safety and other special precautions are being taken than for any other train in history.
>
> Curves are taken slowly. The maximum speed is 45 miles per hour.[3]

The hospital cars seemed to be like serviceable motels, according to the article:

> The hospital cars have regular hospital beds.
>
> Just before the train pulled out, the first meal was served. The men had bread and butter, boiled ham and cabbage, mashed potatoes, ice cream and biscuits and tea or milk.

Extra ice cream and all the milk they could drink were given to those who asked for it.[4]

The detailed itinerary reassured readers that the patients were well-tended and cared for by personnel in every aspect of their care:

> Supper started about 5 p.m., and this consisted of soup or tomato; juice, rib of beef, boiled potatoes, turnips, apple pie or fruit pudding, tea or milk.
>
> Right after supper, the nurses started giving "evening care," which consists of back rubs, special treatments depending on wounds, and generally making the men snug for the night. Then the men were served cocoa or milk.[5]

The trains' efficiency and attention were also the focus of the article:

> On duty in each of the hospital cars are a medical officer, a nursing sister, a medical corporal and a railway porter. Each car has a small kitchen where cocoa and other light food is prepared, and a dispensary.[6]

As reassuring as such articles of the era were, the reality was that the trains frequently deviated from the script:

doctors and nurses were always short on supplies, or out of them. Infections were rampant. Bombs and gunfire were everywhere. Trains on North American soil fared better than those in Europe, but even then, rationing and low resources were the norm, rather than the exception.

Unlike other technological marvels such as tanks and planes, hospital trains were not usually part of concerted wartime propaganda, though there were exceptions. One such case came from the front page of the *Wilmington Star* on June 6, 1940, with the following caption:

> One of the heroic nurses who cared for the wounded among Allied army escaping across the English Channel from Flanders is pictured being removed to a hospital train after arrival in London. British caption accompanying photo said she was wounded when hospital ship [the HMHS] *Paris* was hit by German air bomb.[7]

The name of the nurse was never mentioned, and the "photograph" was an illustration of a comely and unblemished woman with pristine hair. None of the specific facts needed were presented in the article, making it a narrative to emphasize the power of the trains, and the danger encountered, and the selflessness of the hospital personnel, even if many real-life cases at the time, though less melodramatic, were ignored.

Most times, articles of the era usually showcased young soldiers in battle, but in the earlier phases of the war, nurses also played a pivotal part of the story. Some articles emphasized an almost party-like atmosphere as soldiers returned home, with photographs of revellers laughing and posing for the camera as if it were a red-carpet affair, complete with "apple pie made for [the soldier] by his grandmother," as one August 4, 1941, article revealed to readers.[8]

Once the war was over, so too was most of the coverage of the trains, save for one peculiar postscript article in the June 11, 1945, edition of the *Globe and Mail*:

> [R]ail travel to hospital here on board such an effi-
> cient travelling ward as the beautifully built and
> equipped Canadian National Railways hospital car,
> here reproduced in full size and with plate glass
> substituted for one wall so that the public can walk
> on a raised platform alongside and see every detail
> for themselves.[9]

More than presenting an accurate image of the trains to give an understanding of their purpose, the article reads more like a luxury real estate ad:

> The interior color scheme is white and light green.
> Each of the 28 berths has all the comfortable

bedding, the well-arranged lights, ash trays and the like that make over-night travel luxurious on up-to-date trains, but there are extra personal property bags and extra individual comforts for every man, as well as special features affecting the whole car. There's a signal system, of course, with connection to each bunk; there are cupboards full of fresh linens, there's a special entrance for stretchers; there a diet kitchen intended only for the preparation of snacks and special dishes, for each hospital train has its own dining car where regular meals are cooked. The diet kitchen has padding, too, to cut down the noise of silver and crockery in motion. And one woman, looking at the daintily set trays on one or two of the bunks, said as we passed: "They wouldn't have silver like that, of course." But they do, indeed, have shining individual cream jugs, sugar bowls, and little teapots, just "like that." Everything shown is the actual equipment.[10]

There was only one passing mention of those who worked on those trains, but framed as if they were attentive staff at a vacation resort:

But equipment and transportation, we were reminded, are not all—every ambulance train requires a staff of men and women who are trained to work swiftly, skillfully and gently for the comfort and well-being of these wounded boys who are coming home.[11]

Whatever strides and breakthroughs nurses and doctors made suddenly became forgotten, and the trains were repurposed as their historic place was seen as unimportant. While hospital trains were still in use as late as the 1950s during Operation Little Switch in the Korean War (they were described as "splendidly equipped"), their prominence would no longer reach the same levels, nor did the press seem to notice them any longer.[12] How nurses cared for the walking wounded was never mentioned, revered, nor honoured: it was all about the posh creamers and linen, with the author of one article haughtily offended by one observer's questioning of the overly pristine presentation of the train. This was only the beginning of things to come.

What remained was a vague notion that the trains were just a quaint footnote to the epilogue of the hero's journey. The fall from saviour to cab ride home is a shocking development in the history of the trains, but the reality was that the emotional connection was eventually lost to the sands of time. One US pilot recalled his experience of the last days of the war in an article in *World War II* magazine in 2019:

The next four days—May 7-10—were a blur of transit, camps, and delousing showers. During that time, the war had ended—though we didn't know that through any big announcement, but through a gradual awareness that something had changed.

On we went, traveling this time on a hospital train to Camp Lucky Strike at Saint Valery, France. We were told that we would quickly be on a ship sailing back to the good old USA. I wrote a V-mail to Betts and my family: I'm alive. I'm O.K. For me the war is over, and I'm on the way home to get married.[13]

The trains may have saved lives and formed bonds, yet creating memories in the collective became elusive. For many, it was the way to get home from war and then start life over in peace. In Canada, at least, there was a distinctive social and bonding factor in play with hospital trains—after all, these weren't the ones in the thick of a death match; they were the ones who gingerly brought the wounded soldiers home. Many had ridden on the trains in Europe, and now they were transported to be reunited with their loved ones on familiar soil. As one November 18, 1944, *Globe and Mail* article noted, "soldiers who know what it's like to come home on a hospital train often stop to watch their fellow fighting men return on subsequent trains with a patch over a shattered eye, a missing leg, or an empty sleeve."[14] As so many young men returned physically broken, there was some solace in watching the trains bring more compatriots back home, as well as a need to take a second look as a reminder that what had happened on another continent was real. Yet within a year, the trains became a quick carnival side-show or open house before they were brushed aside for a new era of the global village. As far as the press was concerned, the trains had outlived their usefulness as a news peg.

Occasionally, the trains made their way into literature, inspired by the writers' experiences of riding in them. In her book *Chapaev and His Comrades: War and the Russian Literary Hero across the Twentieth Century*, Angela Brintlinger describes one writer's story:

> Vera Panova, a dramatist and novelist who was born in Central Russia, worked off and on as a radio and newspaper journalist and as a copy editor before and during the war, and it was in her role as a journalist that she ended up in the war zone. Initially her assignment had her investigating a military hospital train to produce a propaganda piece about it. As she did this, she met and interviewed dozens of military personnel and got to know their stories. In the end, she finished her piece on the hospital train too late in the war to have it contribute to the

war effort. But she also transformed the characters she met and the experiences she had on the train into fiction for her novel *The Train Companions*.[15]

The reality of those who worked on the hospital trains upset Panova as she was a witness to the death and despair the trains were built to confront:

In December of 1944, Vera Panova left her Perm newspaper (called, coincidentally, *The Star*) and began her life on a military hospital train, where she was charged with the task of writing about the train for a Sanitary Bureau brochure. The experience of train travel in wartime sharpened the experience of war itself. Both aspects of war— waiting around endlessly and being thrown into frenetic activity—are present in this experience and traumatize the passenger just as they do the soldier in the trenches: the long, unnerving waiting and preparing for action and the sudden, overwhelming, and all-consuming activity of dealing with wounded and dying soldiers and civilians. On the one hand, a journey, living and travelling in the train along railroad tracks that had been laid many decades before. On the other hand, the opposite of a journey.[16]

For Panova, the idealism of the trains ultimately became the backbone of her fictional work:

> As Panova relates the conditions in this particular hospital train (and metonymically in wartime itself) she focuses almost entirely on the collective. In fact, her fictional train functions as an ideal work collective, and none of the characters on it assume the role of heroic individual. The very cleanliness of the train was for her a metaphor.[17]

The contributions of those who worked to create the trains and save lives on them were quickly forgotten. The history books favoured stories of soldiers over those of doctors, nurses, cooks, and conductors, who had to scramble to get medication and supplies, and had to make shattered bodies as whole as they could be. Babies were delivered, amputations were performed, and disease had to be staved off. The oversight was disrespectful, and yet few complained. The bottom line was that war was over, but in this case, it was not the secret victors who wrote the history books. The limelight was reserved for soldiers and politicians; there were no accolades for those medical workers who worked and lived on trains.

12

THE LEGACY

IN A MODERN WORLD, HOSPITAL trains seem almost like a forgotten curiosity long left behind, if they are recalled at all. For many people, it is an unknown concept, and not one we often see depicted in period films or documentaries. With different kinds of medical technologies upstaging the very trains that had once been seen as cutting-edge, the mystique could no longer capture the public's imagination. In many ways, the trains were a symbol of power during times of chaos and war; once the Second World War was over, that symbol could no longer exert a psychological pull on those who sought to move on from the past.

Nevertheless, hospital trains, which saved the lives of thousands and altered the fortunes of millions, still left their mark on the scaffolding of modern healthcare, and although their legacy is silent, it is definitive. Despite the dangers, those women and men who worked on the trains felt autonomy and repeatedly made successful life-and-death decisions, paving the way, especially, for future generations of women to progress through mundane stationary hospitals in times of peace. Those who were subsequently confined to the domestic sphere after their service often forgot their lofty contributions or their groundbreaking decisions that saved thousands of lives in a short span of time.

However, these women not only left their collective mark on modern history but sowed the seeds of change in the twentieth century. If one group of women could be effective under the worst possible conditions on a train, with few supplies and an overload of stress and duties, then they could be even more effective in the best conditions during peace. Still, it would take decades before the results of those sown seeds would blossom, making it clear that women could successfully do life-and-death work both on and off the battlefield. Even then, those who worked on the trains never received the credit due to them; they should have been celebrated for how they helped those on the verge of death.

After the war, the trains were divvied up by various interests in the US, while others were acquired by the Ringling Brothers Circus, though one train had a more fitting postwar history as the *Star Presidian* noted on September 18, 1953:

The most unusual Army veteran of World War II has been recalled to duty at Walter Reed Army Medical Center here. A hospital train—"decorated" with campaign ribbons and a battle star for the action in Europe—now is a school-room for medical technicians, pharmacists, ward masters, mess stewards, cooks and clerks. The train has eight ward cars equipped to carry 240 casualties, one dining room-pharmacy car, three cars used for train-staff quarters, and a car to provide power for the entire train. Known as the Third Hospital Train during World War II, it transported more than 33,000 patients over 33,265 between frontlines and rear hospital areas in Europe.[1]

Despite the aforementioned exception, postwar opportunities to use the trains had been lost time and again. Hospital ships seemed grander and more exotic; even today, there are mercy ships for those in medical need without access to traditional hospitals, usually in Africa, though their profile re-emerged during the COVID-19 pandemic, but to a much smaller degree than their heyday.[2] Navies still use hospital ships, usually for disaster relief,[3] and the US Navy plans to unveil a new hospital ship in 2028. Hospital trains, however—dormant until being brought back in Ukraine in 2022—lack sufficient recognition.

This oversight need not continue. A wealth of information slumbers within them, and there are far more puzzle pieces of the past to be gleaned. Hospital trains were thriving ecosystems on their own. Many nations had them, yet they all had very different understandings of what they meant. They were once a sign of a nation's embrace of a technological future and their drive to save their own citizens from slaughter.

It did not matter what side of the dividing line those who were saved by them came from—they were simply grateful to regain their health. Trains raced to intervene and negotiate with death, and those who were picked up by staff came from any of the warring factions. In the end, people are people. As the *National Geographic* noted in one February 2005 article, it was a game of roulette, and anyone's fortunes could be turned around:

One of the wounded soldiers who managed to get on Steuben was Gerhard Dopke. Today a retired teacher, he'd trained as a pilot in the German Luftwaffe until fuel shortages had forced planes to spend most of the time sitting in hangars. Then he'd been sent to join the ground forces, ending up with the Hermann Goring division on the eastern front, where he'd found "mud, hunger, and death."

In late January 1945, Dopke was severely wounded in the head and arm by an exploding grenade. "I had 30 pieces in my body. I was semiconscious when I was transported through Konigsberg (Kaliningrad) to Pillau in a hospital train," he recalls. There he was taken aboard Steuben on a stretcher. "The severely wounded were placed on the upper decks," he says, "and that saved me."[4]

Those who remember the trains understand their legacy as saviours that gave the gift of a precious second chance. The mandate of the trains was peace and survival. In the end, the medical staff on the trains beat even the soldiers in their longevity: those who fought with guns eventually stopped firing and put down their weapons, whereas those who healed them carried on long after the battles ended. Even after the war, former hospital train doctors and nurses would be greeted over the years by the very soldiers they rescued just to be told *thank you*.

Though the trains were a crucial part of the war effort, until now, history still forgets how central they were to the Allied mythos, and to Europe's survival. They were more powerful than tanks or bombs, and they broke barriers as they raced to the rescue of war victims and facilitated the healing of torn flesh and shattered limbs. The dividing lines of war were crossed by those trains as friendships were seeded and blossomed. Those who worked on the trains were not just the nurses and doctors of a mere city, but of an entire continent, united in the battle against death, all with limited supplies as they were targeted by gunfire from those they often would rescue and heal.

The peculiar logic of the trains is an enigma the modern world has yet to ponder in earnest. What lessons can be learned? How can we see their influence on current affairs?

Perhaps the greatest lesson is the most challenging to accept: what was once central to survival can be easily forgotten. We can be frightened and believe that no one will be there for us, and yet the hospital trains and the mentality held by those who worked within them demonstrates the triumph of the human spirit: we will race to those who need us, even when we face danger and lack the most basic tools to solve the problem—but solve it we will.

While it is true that the central lesson in one era can be easily forgotten in another, we can look back to the past at any time of our choosing and rediscover what we forgot—or discover something we had no idea ever existed. There are hints that the trains may be revived during times of conflict. Some nations have various forms of hospital trains, including Mexico, Russia, Malta, South Africa, India, and China. Some trains are now seeing combat, as the *Globe and Mail* reported on April 15, 2022:

> Dr. Liu arrived in Ukraine in the last week of March as part of an emergency response team.

She travelled to eastern parts of the country, where Doctors Without Borders has used a specially equipped train to evacuate people from areas that have seen fierce fighting. The rolling medical facility, a modern-day echo of hospital trains used in the Second World War and earlier conflicts, has allowed doctors to reach into the country's disputed Donbas region.

Doctors Without Borders has used the train, which has modified sleeper cars as patient rooms, to transport about 300 people to safety in western Ukraine, Dr. Liu said. Ukrainian Railways has begun operating its trains at slow speeds to limit injuries in case they are struck by Russian forces, she added.[5]

People can be brilliant, innovative, resilient, loving, brave, patient, and idealistic all at the same time. We are independent and individualistic, and we can rise to the challenge of any crisis. We can come together when everything falls apart. We've seen this not just on the battlefields but also on the hospital trains, where the broken were put back together and given another day, another chance. Those who survived, thanks to those who rode on a different track, could see the power of those trains: the nurses who rallied the injured and showed them humanity, and the doctors who fixed them under fire.

In a modern world where peace seems to be threatened, the hospital trains of the Second World War serve as an antidote to helplessness and despair, and are a powerful reminder that no threat can withstand the benevolence of the human spirit. No one should ever be ruled by fear, but kindness, bravery, love, truth and optimism. Those qualities made those who worked on those trains the most valuable players of the war—especially the ones who did so quietly, diligently, and most of all, humbly.

ACKNOWLEDGEMENTS

I WOULD LIKE TO THANK Dushica Puharic, Gerhard and Hettie Greeve, David Neace, the World War II US Medical Research Center, and the Imperial War Museum for their cooperation on this book.

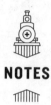

NOTES

[1] In Chaos, There is Order

1. "History of military hospital trains in the Second World War. Railway medical transport," (*Mstone*, mstone-ru. com, undated).

2. Medical Society of Delaware, *Delaware State Medical Journal*, vol. 16, iss. 1 (January 1944). https://archive. org/details/sim_delaware-medical-journal_1944-01_16_1.

3. "Pioneer Hospital Train Worker Tells of her First Trip," *The Fog Horn (Letterman General Hospital)*, vol. 4 (October 14, 1944): 2.

4. "First Overseas-Type Army Hospital Train To Be Exhibited Here," *Washington Evening Star* (November 22, 1943): B4.

5. Frank Gervasi, "Hospital Train," *Washington Evening Star*, January 18, 1942: 14.

6. Ibid.

7.   Meyer Berger, (1943). "Hope Reborn in Wounded As
     Hospital Train Goes West; Soldiers From Salerno,
     Sicily and Africa Quit East for Treatment Nearer
     Home at Yuletide and Aches Are Forgotten; HOPE IS
     BORN ANEW ON HOSPITAL TRAIN THE BEST WE
     HAVE IS HELD NONE TOO GOOD FOR THESE,"
     New York Times, December 13, 1943: 1. https://www.
     nytimes.com/1943/12/13/archives/hope-reborn-in-
     wounded-as-hospital-train-goes-west-soldiers-from.
     html?smid=url-share.

8.   "Army Hospital Train Will Be Used During Summer
     Maneuvers," *Washington Evening Star*, May 19, 1941: B2.

9.   "Pvt. John Shepherd On Navy Hospital Train,"
     Lexington Advertiser, May 3, 1945: 4.

10. "Durant Boy Member of Hospital Train That Cares
     For Wounded Soldiers: Capt. John B. Wilkes Transfers
     Wounded From Battle Action," *The Durant News*, July 6,
     1944: 1.

11. US Army, *Bulletin of the United States Army Medical
     Department*, no. 72 (January 1944).

12. "'Ike' salutes war wounded as train leaves for capital,"
     Los Angeles Daily News, June 25, 1945: 4.

[2] A Brief History of Hospital Trains

1.   Michael Foley, *Britain›s Railways in the Second World
     War* (Barnsley, UK: Pen and Sword Transport, 2021).

2.   Markus Figl and Linda E. Pelinka, "Jaromir Baron
     von Mundy—Founder of the Vienna ambulance ser-
     vice," *Resuscitation*, vol. 66, iss. 2 (August 2005):
     121–25, https://doi.org/10.1016/j.resuscitation.2005.03.004.

3. Ibid.

4. "Tenth Ohio's Sick," *Maysville Evening Bulletin*, September 5, 1898: 1.

5. "Ohio's Hospital Train," *Maysville Evening Bulletin*, September 5, 1989: 1.

6. Ibid.

7. "A Kentucky Hospital Camp Train," *Indianapolis Journal*, September 2, 1898: 2.

8. "Health of the Army," *Hope Pioneer*, December 8, 1898: 4.

9. Alan J. Hawk, "An ambulating hospital: or, how the hospital train transformed Army medicine," *Civil War History*, vol. 48, no. 3 (2002): 197–219.

10. "A Protest from the Thunderer," *Globe and Mail*, July 16, 1904: 22.

11. William Marchington, "Lady Charles Ross on Hospital Train," *Toronto Globe*, January 7, 1915: 1.

12. "War Summary," *Globe and Mail*, March 9, 1917: 1.

13. Associated Press, "Army Hospital Train Carries First Load," *Tonopah Daily Bonanza*, January 26, 1917: 1.

14. Ibid.

15. Ibid.

16. "New American Hospital Train for France," *Hanford Daily Journal*, June 8, 1918: 1.

17. Associated Press, "Hospital Train Given France by Americans," San José Mercury-News, February 15, 1916: 5.

18. J.D.C. Bennett, "Princess Vera Gedroits: military surgeon, poet, and author," *British Medical Journal*, vol. 305, no. 6868 (December 19, 1992): 1532. https://doi.org/10.1136/bmj.305.6868.1532.

19. Ibid.

20. Medical Society of Delaware, *Delaware State Medical Journal*, vol. 16, iss. 1 (January 1944).

21. Ibid.

22. Ibid.

23. "900 Yanks Freed; Arrive in France," *Washington Times*, December 1, 1918: 1.

[3] The Evolution of Hospital Trains

1. Clarence McKittrick Smith, *The Medical Department: Hospitalization and Evacuation, Zone of Interior*, vol. 1 (Washington, DC: US Army, Office of the Chief of Military History, 1956), https://history.army.mil/html/books/010/10-7/index.html.

2. Michael T. Fleming, "United States Army Hospital Trains," *The Timetable* (August 2015), https://www.nmra.org.

3. "Rail Death Smash Toll Set at 80," *Globe and Mail*, December 26, 1938: 1.

4. Nicola Tyrer, *Sisters in Arms: British Army Nurses Tell Their Story* (London: Weidenfeld & Nicolson Ltd., 2008).

5. C.M. Smith, *The Medical Department: Hospitalization and Evacuation, Zone of Interior*, vol. 1 (Washington, DC: US Army, Office of the Chief of Military History, 1956).

6. G.H. Bennett, *Destination Normandy: Three American Regiments on D-Day* (Mechanicsburg, PA: Stackpole Books, 2009).

7. Chester Wardlow, *The Transportation Corps: Movements, Training, and Supply*, vol. 2 (Washington, DC: US Army, Office of the Chief of Military History, 1956).

8. R.H.B. Dear, "Medico-Military Aspects of the Repatriation of Sick and Wounded," *Military Surgeon*, vol. 105, iss. 1 (1949): 64-71.

9. C.M. Smith, *The Medical Department: Hospitalization and Evacuation, Zone of Interior*, vol. 1 (Washington, DC: US Army, Office of the Chief of Military History, 1956).

10. Ibid.

11. "Hundreds Here Visit 10-car Hospital Train Displayed by Army," *Washington Evening Star*, November 25, 1943: B1.

12. Ibid.

[4] The Trains of the Second World War

1. US Army, European Theater of Operations, *That Men Might Live!: The Story of the Medical Service—ETO*, G.I. Stories of the Ground, Air and Service Forces in the European Theater of Operations (Paris: Dupont, 1945); accessed via the University of Alabama Libraries Special Collections, 1945, Box: 1, Folder: 43., PM-016. http://archives.lib.ua.edu/repositories/3/archival_objects/199263.

2. C.M. Smith, *The Medical Department: Hospitalization and Evacuation, Zone of Interior*, vol. 1 (Washington, DC: US Army, Office of the Chief of Military History, 1956).

3.   Ibid.

4.   Larry K. Neal Jr., "Railroads Carry Wounded
      Soldiers," *World War II, 1941 (1945)*: 15.

5.   *Evacuation, Zone of Interior*, vol. 1 (Washington, DC:
      US Army, Office of the Chief of Military History, 1956).

6.   Ibid.

7.   Larry K. Neal Jr., "Railroads Carry Wounded
      Soldiers," *World War II, 1941 (1945)*: 15.

8.   C.M. Smith, *The Medical Department: Hospitalization
      and Evacuation, Zone of Interior*, vol. 1 (Washington, DC:
      US Army, Office of the Chief of Military History, 1956).

9.   Ibid.

10.   Ibid.

11.   R. Tourret, *Allied Military Locomotives of the Second
      World War: War Department Locomotives* (Abingdon,
      UK: Tourret Publishing, 1976).

12.   Michael T. Fleming, "United States Army Hospital Trains,"
      The Timetable (August 2015), https://www.nmra.org.

13.   C.M. Smith, *The Medical Department: Hospitalization
      and Evacuation, Zone of Interior*, vol. 1 (Washington, DC:
      US Army, Office of the Chief of Military History, 1956).

14.   Ibid.

15.   "War Discards Used for Hospital Train." *Globe and
      Mail*, December 3, 1943: 7.

16.   "Smiles, Tears, Cheers Greet First Hospital Train; 86
      Homecomers Disperse to Homes, Institutions," *Globe
      and Mail*, November 29, 1943: 15.

17. Ibid.

18. "No Hospital Train Yet," *Adelaide News*, August 29, 1941: 8.

19. "Hospital Train Built for Military," *Barrier Miner*, February 5, 1942: 2.

20. Photo caption, *Adelaide News*, March 10, 1942: 3.

21. Photo caption, *Central Queensland Herald*, March 19, 1942: 19.

22. "Second Group of Wounded Leave," *Lethbridge Herald*, January 6, 1944: 5.

23. C.M. Smith, *The Medical Department: Hospitalization and Evacuation, Zone of Interior*, vol. 1 (Washington, DC: US Army, Office of the Chief of Military History, 1956).

24. World War II US Medical Research Center, "The Hospital Train in the E.T.O. 1944–1945," undated, https://www.med-dept.com/articles/the-hospital-train-in-the-e-t-o-1944-1945/.

25. R. Tourret, *Allied Military Locomotives of the Second World War: War Department Locomotives* (Abingdon, UK: Tourret Publishing, 1976).

[5] The Nurses

1. Kathi Jackson, *They Called Them Angels: American Military Nurses of World War II* (Lincoln, NE: University of Nebraska Press, 2006).

2. Cynthia Toman, "Front Lines and Frontiers: War as 2. Legitimate Work for Nurses, 1939–1945," *Histoire sociale/Social History*, vol. 40, no. 79 (2007).

3.   "Army Hospital Trains," *The American Journal of Nursing* 43, no. 6 (1943): 565–66. https://doi.org/10.2307/3416358.

4.   Diane Burke Fessler, *No Time for Fear: Voices of American Military Nurses in World War II* (East Lansing, MI: Michigan State University Press, 1996).

5.   Ibid.

6.   Sean C.W. Korsgaard, "'You are going to make it home': 96-year-old Army nurse recalls time healing our heroes." *The Progress-Index*, September 8, 2016, https://www.progress-index.com/story/news/2016/09/08/you-are-going-to/25491174007/.

7.   Ibid.

8.   Ibid.

9.   Eric Taylor, *Wartime Nurse: One Hundred Years from the Crimea to Korea, 1854–1954* (London: Isis Large Print Books, 2002).

[6] **The Doctors**

1.   "Troops Praise Army Doctors," *Globe and Mail*, November 27, 1943: 18.

2.   William R. Feasby, *Official History of the Canadian Medical Services, 1939–1945: Volume 1, Organization and Campaigns*, Department of National Defense (Ottawa: Queen's Printer, 1956).

3.   B.M. Bosworth, "Splints and casts in the treatment of war injuries," *The American Journal of Surgery*, vol. 72, no. 3 (1946): 385–92, https://doi.org/10.1016/0002-9610(46)90328-5.

4. M. Bak, "Kórházvonatos tapasztalatok a II. világháború fertözö betegségeiröl" [Experience with hospital trains with regard to transmissible diseases during World War II], *Orvosi Hetilap*, vol. 124 no. 42 (1983): 2568–70.

5. Ibid.

6. Ibid.

7. Ibid.

8. Ibid.

9. Stanley Aylett, *Surgeon at War 1939–45: The Second World War Seen from Operating Tables Behind the Front Line* (London: Metro Books, 2015).

[7] The Patients

1. Associated Press, "War-Maimed Find Army Merciful; Helps Smooth 'Road Back,'" *Oakland Tribune*, December 13, 1943: 4.

2. E.H. Botterell, A.T. Jousse, C. Aberhart, and J.W. Cluff, "Paraplegia following war," *Canadian Medical Association Journal*, 55(3) (1946): 249.

3. Kathy Uek, "Former workers, patients remember hospital created for WWII service members," *The Repository*, July 28, 2009, https://www.cantonrep. com/story/news/2009/07/28/former-workers-patients-remember-hospital/47936441007/.

4. Photo caption, *Hillston Spectator and Lachlan River Advertiser*, August 16, 1945: 1.

5. "Army Patients Moved," *Sausalito News*, May 17, 1945: 4.

6.   "Veterans Arrive In First Hospital Train To Bring
      Casualties," *Globe and Mail*, August 4, 1941: 4.

7.   Ibid.

8.   "Walking Wounded Back From Italy and England,"
      Globe and Mail, March 27, 1944: 5.

9.   "Two UFFO Members Die," *The Fisherman*, February 16,
      1945: 2.

10.   William R. Feasby, *Official History of the Canadian
      Medical Services, 1939–1945: Volume 1, Organization
      and Campaigns*, Department of National Defense
      (Ottawa: Queen's Printer, 1956).

[8] The Battles

1.   "History of military hospital trains in the Second World
      War. Railway medical transport," (*Mstone*, mstone-ru.
      com, undated).

2.   Lynn Heinzerling, "Russia loses many troops in big
      battle," *Wilmington Morning Star*, January 1, 1940: 1.

3.   Harold Denny, "WIN MAJOR VICTORY—Vast War
      Booty Seized as Russians Flee in Two Defeats SOVIET
      WIDENS AIR RAIDS—Civilians Victims, Hospital Hit
      in Dozen Bomb Attacks, Some at Undefended Points."
      New York Times, January 1, 1940: 1.

4.   "Editorial: USA Army Medical Report (1940)," *BMJ
      Military Health*, vol. 77, no. 1 (July 1941): 37–39,
      https://militaryhcalth.bmj.com/content/77/1/37.

5.   Charles M. Walson, "Some of the Medical
      Accomplishments in New York, New Jersey, and
      Delaware during World War II with Particular

Reference to Metropolitan New York," *Military Surgeon*, vol. 100, iss. 4 (April 1947): 294-305, https://doi.org/10.1093/milmed/100.4.294.

6.   Michael Foley, *Britain's Railways in the Second World War* (Barnsley, UK: Pen and Sword Transport, 2021).

7.   Cynthia Toman, *An Officer and a Lady: Canadian Military Nursing and the Second World War* (Vancouver: UBC Press, 2007), p. 50.

8.   Photo caption, *West Australian*, June 11, 1940: 10.

9.   J.L.S. Coulter, *The Royal Naval Medical Service, Vol. II: Operations*, History of the Second World War: United Kingdom Medical Series (London: HM Stationery Office, 1954).

10.   Nicola Tyrer, *Sisters in Arms: British Army Nurses Tell Their Story* (London: Weidenfeld & Nicolson Ltd., 2008).

11.   US Army, European Theater of Operations, *That Men Might Live!: The Story of the Medical Service—ETO*, G.I. Stories of the Ground, Air and Service Forces in the European Theater of Operations (Paris: Dupont, 1945); accessed via the University of Alabama Libraries Special Collections, 1945, Box: 1, Folder: 43., PM-016. http://archives.lib.ua.edu/repositories/3/archival_objects/199263.

12.   Leonard D. Heaton, *Annual Report of the Surgeon General, US Army* (Washington, DC: Office of the Surgeon General, 1961).

13.   James Hayward, *Myths & Legends of the Second World War* (Cheltenham, UK: History Press, 2009).

14. Michael Foley, *Britain's Railways in the Second World War* (Barnsley, UK: Pen and Sword Transport, 2021).

15. Lindsay J. Morgan, H. Morgan, and B. Morgan, "Notes from a War Diary—The Isle of Wight and Tripoli," *BMJ Military Health: Journal of the Royal Army Medical Corps*, vol. 156, no. 1 (March 2010): 73-74, https://doi.org/10.1136/jramc-156-01-19.

16. Ibid.

17. Ibid.

18. "State vets admitted to Foster General," *Mississippi Enterprise*, July 1, 1944:1.

[9] The Future is Past

1. US Army, European Theater of Operations, *That Men Might Live!: The Story of the Medical Service—ETO*, G.I. Stories of the Ground, Air and Service Forces in the European Theater of Operations (Paris: Dupont, 1945); accessed via the University of Alabama Libraries Special Collections, 1945, Box: 1, Folder: 43., PM-016. http://archives.lib.ua.edu/repositories/3/archival_objects/199263.

2. Ibid.

3. Ibid.

4. Oscar Paul Dost, "What the United States of America Did for the Railway Transportation of the Sick," trans. Claudius F. Mayer, *Military Medicine*, vol. 119, iss. 4 (October 1956): 250–52, https://doi.org/10.1093/milmed/119.4.250.

5. Ibid.

6.   Ibid.

7.   John Hedley-Whyte and Debra R. Milamed, "Surgical
      Travellers: Tapestry to Bayeux." *The Ulster Medical
      Journal* 83, no. 3 (June 2014): 171–77, http://nrs.
      harvard.edu/urn-3:HUL.InstRepos:22423612.

8.   Joseph R. Darnall, "Fixed Hospital Reconnaissance
      on the Western Front in the Fall of 1944," *Military
      Surgeon*, vol. 103, iss. 4 (October 1948): 251–60,
      https://doi.org/10.1093/milmed/103.4.251.

9.   Ibid.

[10] The Secret Social

1.   Jane Brooks, "Reasserting work, space and gender
      boundaries at the end of the Second World War," in
      *Negotiating Nursing: British Army Sisters and Soldiers
      in the Second World War* (Manchester: Manchester
      University Press, 2019): 168–98, https://doi.org/10.77
      65/9781526147257.00012.

2.   "They'll Never Die: WWII and the Eternal Legacy
      of our Grandfathers," *Russia Beyond*, May 9, 2016,
      https://www.rbth.com/arts/history/2016/05/09/
      theyll-never-die-wwii-and-the-eternal-legacy-of-our-
      grandfathers_591313.

3.   Lorna F. Laffer, "I Worked on a Hospital Train:
      Experiences of a Nurse Working on a Northern
      Territory Ambulance Train in World War 2," reprinted
      from *Australasian Nurses Journal, Northern Perspective*
      18, no. 2 (January 1995): 74–79.

4.   "Druggists have April Bond Drive; La Jolla Druggists
     ask you to buy war bonds from them during April," *La
     Jolla Journal*, April 6, 1944: 1.

5.   "Local Druggists Join Move to Buy Hospital Train," *La
     Jolla Light*, April 13, 1944: 1.

6.   Bob Carruthers, *Servants of Evil: New First-Hand
     Accounts of the Second World War from Survivors of
     Hitler's Armed Forces* (Minneapolis: Zenith Press,
     2004).

7.   Ibid.

[II] The Image

1.   "Soldier on Hospital Train Cheered by Fiancée's
     Welcome," *Globe and Mail*, June 26, 1944: 4.

2.   "Throng Cheers Veterans Home from War Zones,"
     Globe and Mail, April 15, 1944: 4.

3.   "Hospital Train Unique from Safety Standpoint," *Globe
     and Mail*, November 26, 1943: 2.

4.   Ibid.

5.   Ibid.

6.   Ibid.

7.   Photo caption, *Wilmington Morning Star*, June 6, 1940: 1.

8.   Veterans Arrive in First Hospital Train to Bring
     Casualties, *Globe and Mail*, August 4, 1941: 4.

9.   "The Homemaker: HOSPITAL ON WHEELS," *Globe
     and Mail*, June 11, 1945: 13.

10.   Ibid.

11.   Ibid.

12.   World War II US Medical Research Center, "The Hospital Train in the E.T.O. 1944–1945," undated, https://www.med-dept.com/articles/the-hospital-train-in-the-e-t-o-1944-1945/.

13.   Richard A. Gray, "Down But Not Out: A Pilot Describes the Bad Luck—And a Lot of Good—He Encountered in the Final Month of the War," *World War II*, vol. 33, no. 5 (February 2019): 38.

14.   "Beribboned Sergeant Says Army Like Team," *Globe and Mail*, November 18, 1944: 4.

15.   Angela Brintlinger, *Chapaev and His Comrades: War and the Russian Literary Hero Across the Twentieth Century* (Brookline, MA: Academic Studies Press, 2012).

16.   Ibid.

17.   Ibid.

[12] The Legacy

1.   "Army 'Big Train' Given Chance to Serve Once More," *Star Presidian*, September 18, 1953: 3.

2.   Gidget Fuentes, "Hospital Ship *Comfort* Ends NYC COVID-19 Mission After Treating 182 Patients," *USNI News*, April 27, 2020, https://news.usni.org/2020/04/27/hospital-ship-comfort-ends-nyc-covid-19-mission-after-treating-182-patients.

3. Michael Schwirtz, "The 1,000-Bed *Comfort* Was Supposed to Aid New York. It Has 20 Patients," *New York Times*, April 2, 2020, https://www.nytimes.com/2020/04/02/nyregion/ny-coronavirus-usns-comfort.html.

4. Marcin Jamkowski, "Ghost Ship Found: As World War II Neared Its Bloody Finale, the Red Army Stormed into East Prussia." *National Geographic*, vol. 207, no. 2 (February 2005): 32–51.

5. Nathan Vanderklippe, "Canada is failing Ukrainians displaced by Russian invasion, former head of Doctors Without Borders says." *Globe and Mail*, April 15, 2022, https://www.theglobeandmail.com/world/article-canada-is-failing-ukrainians-displaced-by-russian-invasion-former-head/.

BIBLIOGRAPHY

"Army Hospital Trains." *American Journal of Nursing* 43, no. 6 (1943): 565–66. https://doi.org/10.2307/3416358.

"Editorial: USA Army Medical Report (1940)." *BMJ Military Health*, vol. 77, no. 1 (July 1941): 37–39, https://military-health.bmj.com/content/77/1/37.

"Pioneer Hospital Train Worker Tells of her First Trip." *The Fog Horn* (Letterman General Hospital), vol. 4 (October 14, 1944).

Adelaide News. "No Hospital Train Yet." August 29, 1941.

———. Photo caption. March 10, 1942.

Altman, Howard. "The Navy's First Medical Ship In 35 Years Will Be Unlike Any Before It." *The War Zone.* April 29, 2022. https://www.thedrive.com/the-war-zone/the-navys-first-medical-ship-in-35-years-will-be-unlike-any-before-it.

Associated Press. "Hospital Train Given France by Americans." *San José Mercury-News*, February 15, 1916.

Aylett, Stanley. (2015). *Surgeon at War 1939–45: The Second World War Seen from Operating Tables Behind the Front Line.* London: Metro Books, 2015.

Bak, M. "Kórházvonatos tapasztalatok a II. világháború fertözö betegségeiröl" [Experience with hospital trains with regard to transmissible diseases during World War II]. *Orvosi Hetilap*, vol. 124, no. 42 (1983): 2568-70.

Barrier Miner. "Hospital Train Built for Military." February 5, 1942.

Bellafaire, Judith A. "The Army Nurse Corps: A Commemoration of World War II Service." *CMH Pub* no. 72-14. Washington, DC: US Army Center of Military History, 1993.

Bennett, G.H. *Destination Normandy: Three American Regiments on D-Day.* Mechanicsburg, PA: Stackpole Books, 2009.

Bennett, J.D.C. "Princess Vera Gedroits: military surgeon, poet, and author," *British Medical Journal*, vol. 305, no. 6868 (December 19, 1992): 1532. https://doi.org/10.1136/bmj.305.6868.1532.

Berger, Meyer. "Hope Reborn in Wounded As Hospital Train Goes West; Soldiers From Salerno, Sicily and Africa Quit East for Treatment Nearer Home at Yuletide and Aches Are Forgotten; HOPE IS BORN ANEW ON HOSPITAL TRAIN THE BEST WE HAVE IS HELD NONE TOO GOOD FOR THESE." *New York Times.* December 13, 1943.

Bosworth, B.M. (1946). "Splints and casts in the treatment of war injuries." *The American Journal of Surgery*, vol. 72, no. 3 (1946): 385-92. https://doi.org/10.1016/0002-9610(46)90328-5.

Botterell, E.H., A.T. Jousse, C. Aberhart, and J.W. Cluff, (1946). "Paraplegia following war." *Canadian Medical Association Journal*, 55(3) (1946): 249

Brintlinger, Angela. *Chapaev and His Comrades: War and the Russian Literary Hero Across the Twentieth Century.* Brookline, MA: Academic Studies Press, 2012.

Brooks, Jane. "Reasserting work, space and gender boundaries at the end of the Second World War." In *Negotiating Nursing: British Army Sisters and Soldiers in the Second World War* (Manchester: Manchester University Press, 2019): 168–98. https://doi.org/10.7765/9781526147257.00012

Burke Fessler, Diane. *No Time for Fear: Voices of American Military Nurses in World War II*. East Lansing, MI: Michigan State University Press, 1996.

Carruthers, Bob. *Servants of Evil: New First-Hand Accounts of the Second World War from Survivors of Hitler's Armed Forces*. Minneapolis: Zenith Press, 2004.

Central Queensland Herald. Photo caption. March 19, 1942.

Coulter, J.L.S. *The Royal Naval Medical Service, Vol. I: Administration*. History of the Second World War: United Kingdom Medical Series London: HM Stationery Office, 1954. Royal Naval Medical Service (1954).

———. *The Royal Naval Medical Service, Vol. II: Operations*. History of the Second World War: United Kingdom Medical Series. London: HM Stationery Office, 1954.

Darnall, Joseph R. "Fixed Hospital Reconnaissance on the Western Front in the Fall of 1944." *Military Surgeon*, vol. 103, iss. 4 (October 1948): 251–60. https://doi.org/10.1093/milmed/103.4.251.

Dear, R.H.B. "Medico-Military Aspects of the Repatriation of Sick and Wounded," *Military Surgeon*, vol. 105, iss. 1 (1949): 64–71.

Denny, Harold. "WIN MAJOR VICTORY; Vast War Booty Seized as Russians Flee in Two Defeats SOVIET WIDENS AIR RAIDS Civilians Victims, Hospital Hit in Dozen Bomb Attacks, Some at Undefended Points." *New York Times*. January 1, 1940.

Dost, Oscar Paul. "What the United States of America Did for the Railway Transportation of the Sick." Translated by Claudius F. Mayer. *Military Medicine*, vol. 119, iss. 4 (October 1956): 250–52. https://doi.org/10.1093/milmed/119.4.250

Feasby, W.R. *Official History of the Canadian Medical Services, 1939–1945: Volume 1, Organization and Campaigns*. Department of National Defense. Ottawa: Queen's Printer, 1956.

Figl, Markus and Linda E. Pelinka. "Jaromir Baron von Mundy—Founder of the Vienna ambulance service." *Resuscitation*, vol. 66, iss. 2 (August 2005): 121–25. https://doi.org/10.1016/j.resuscitation.2005.03.004.

Fleming, Michael T. "United States Army Hospital Trains." *The Timetable*. August 2015. https://www.nmra.org.

Foley, Michael. *Britain's Railways in the Second World War.* Barnsley, UK: Pen and Sword Transport, 2021.

Fuentes, Gidget. "Hospital Ship Comfort Ends NYC COVID-19 Mission After Treating 182 Patients." *USNI News*, April 27, 2020. https://news.usni.org/2020/04/27/hospital-ship-comfort-ends-nyc-covid-19-mission-after-treating-182-patients.

Gervasi, Frank. "Hospital Train." *Washington Evening Star.* January 18, 1942.

Globe and Mail. (1917). "War Summary." March 9, 1917.

——. "A Protest from the Thunderer." July 16, 1904.

——. "Beribboned Sergeant Says Army Like Team." November 18, 1944.

——. "Hospital Train Unique From Safety Standpoint." November 26, 1943.

——. "Nazis Taken at Dieppe Well Treated, Say Wounded Men Arriving Home." October 15, 1942.

——. "Rail Death Smash Toll Set at 80." December 26, 1938.

——. "Smiles, Tears, Cheers Greet First Hospital Train; 86 Homecomers Disperse to Homes, Institutions." November 29, 1943.

——. "Soldier on Hospital Train Cheered by Fiancée's Welcome." June 26, 1944.

——. "The Homemaker: HOSPITAL ON WHEELS." June 11, 1945.

——. "Throng Cheers Veterans Home From War Zones." April 15, 1944.

——. "Troops Praise Army Doctors." November 27, 1943.

——. "Veterans Arrive In First Hospital Train To Bring Casualties." August 4, 1941.

——. "Walking Wounded Back From Italy and England." March 27, 1944.

———. "War Discards Used for Hospital Train." December 3, 1943.

Gray, Richard A. "Down But Not Out: A Pilot Describes the Bad Luck—And a Lot of Good—He Encountered in the Final Month of the War." *World War II*, vol. 33, no. 5 (February 2019): 38.

Hanford Daily Journal. "New American Hospital Train for France." June 8, 1918.

Harrison, Ada M. *Grey and Scarlet: Letters from the War Areas by Army Sisters on Active Service*. London: Hodder & Stoughton, 1944.

Hawk, Alan J. "An ambulating hospital: or, how the hospital train transformed Army medicine," *Civil War History*, vol. 48, no. 3 (2002): 197–219.

Hayward, James. *Myths & Legends of the Second World War*. Cheltenham, UK: History Press, 2009.

Heaton, Leonard D. *Annual Report of the Surgeon General, US Army*. Washington, DC: Office of the Surgeon General, 1961.

Hedley-Whyte, John, and Debra R. Milamed. "Surgical Travellers: Tapestry to Bayeux." *Ulster Medical Journal*, vol. 83, no. 3 (June 2014): 171–77. http://nrs.harvard.edu/urn-3:HUL.InstRepos:22423612

Heinzerling, Lynn. "Russia loses many troops in big battle." *Wilmington Morning Star*. January 1, 1940.

Hillston Spectator and Lachlan River Advertiser. Photo caption. August 16, 1945.

Hope Pioneer. "Health of the Army." December 8, 1898.

Horne, Madison. "Women of the WWII Workforce: Photos Show the Real-Life Rosie the Riveters." *History Channel.* June 11, 2019, updated May 11, 2021. https://www.history.com/news/women-world-war-ii-factories-photos.

Hume, Edgar Erskine. "United Nations medical service in Korean conflict." *Journal of the American Medical Association*, vol. 146, no. 14 (August 4, 1951): 1307-10. doi:10.1001/jama.1951.03670140033009.

Indianapolis Journal. "A Kentucky Hospital Camp Train." September 2, 1898.

Jackson, Kathi. *They Called Them Angels: American Military Nurses of World War II*. Lincoln, NE: University of Nebraska Press, 2006.

Jamkowski, Marcin. "Ghost Ship Found: As World War II Neared Its Bloody Finale, the Red Army Stormed into East Prussia." *National Geographic*, vol. 207, no. 2 (February 2005): 32-51.

Korsgaard, Sean C.W. "'You are going to make it home': 96-year-old Army nurse recalls time healing our heroes." *The Progress-Index*. September 8, 2016. https://www.progress-index.com/story/news/2016/09/08/you-are-going-to/25491174007/.

La Jolla Journal. "Druggists have April Bond Drive; La Jolla Druggists ask you to buy war bonds from them during April." April 6, 1944.

La Jolla Light. "Local Druggists Join Move To Buy Hospital Train." April 13, 1944.

Laffer, Lorna. "I Worked on a Hospital Train: Experiences of a Nurse Working on a Northern Territory Ambulance Train in World War 2." Reprinted from *Australasian Nurses Journal. Northern Perspective* 18, no. 2 (January 1995): 74-79.

Lethbridge Herald. "Second Group of Wounded Leave." January 6, 1944.

Lexington Advertiser. "Pvt. John Shepherd On Navy Hospital Train." May 3, 1945.

Los Angeles Daily News. "'Ike' salutes war wounded as train leaves for capital." June 25, 1945.

Major, Susan. *Female Railway Workers in World War II.* Barnsley, UK: Pen & Sword, 2018.

Marchington, William. "Lady Charles Ross on Hospital Train." *Toronto Globe,* January 7, 1915.

Maysville Evening Bulletin. "Ohio's Hospital Train." September 5, 1898.

———. "Tenth Ohio's Sick." September 5, 1898.

McEwen, Yvonne T. (2016). *In the Company of Nurses: The History of the British Army Nursing Service in the Great War.* Edinburgh: Edinburgh University Press, 2014.

McMinn, John H., and Max Levin. (1963). *Personnel in World War II,* Vol. 2. Medical Department, United States Army, in World War II and Administrative series. Washington, DC: Office of the Surgeon General, Dept. of the Army, 1963. http://resource.nlm.nih.gov/1278009R.

Medical Society of Delaware. *Delaware State Medical Journal,* vol. 16, iss. 1 (January 1944). https://archive.org/details/sim_delaware-medical-journal_1944-01_16_1.

Mississippi Enterprise. "State vets admitted to Foster General." July 1, 1944.

Morgan, Lindsay J., H. Morgan, and B. Morgan. "Notes from a War Diary—The Isle of Wight and Tripoli." *BMJ Military Health: Journal of the Royal Army Medical Corps,* vol. 156, no. 1 (March 2010): 73–74. https://doi.org/10.1136/jramc-156-01-19.

Mstone. "History of Military Hospital Trains in the Second World War. Railway Medical Transport." Undated. mstone-ru.com.

Neal Jr., Larry K. "Railroads Carry Wounded Soldiers." *World War II, 1941* (1945): 15.

Oakland Tribune. "War-Maimed Find Army Merciful; Helps Smooth 'Road Back.'" December 13, 1943.

Quinn, Roswell. "Rethinking Antibiotic Research and Development: World War II and the Penicillin Collaborative." *American Journal of Public Health*, vol. 103, iss. 3 (March 2013): 426–34. https://doi.org/10.2105/AJPH.2012.300693

Russia Beyond. "They'll never die: WWII and the eternal legacy of our grandfathers." May 9, 2016. https://www.rbth.com/arts/history/2016/05/09/theyll-never-die-wwii-and-the-eternal-legacy-of-our-grandfathers_591313.

Sausalito News. "Army Patients Moved." May 17, 1945.

Schwirtz, Michael. "The 1,000-Bed *Comfort* Was Supposed to Aid New York. It Has 20 Patients." *New York Times*, April 2, 2020. https://www.nytimes.com/2020/04/02/nyregion/ny-coronavirus-usns-comfort.html.

Smith, Clarence McKittrick. *The Medical Department: Hospitalization and Evacuation, Zone of Interior*, vol. 1 (Washington, DC: US Army, Office of the Chief of Military History, 1956), https://history.army.mil/html/books/010/10-7/index.html.

Star Presidian. "Army 'Big Train' Given Chance to Serve Once More." September 18, 1953.

Taylor, Eric. *Wartime Nurse: One Hundred Years from the Crimea to Korea, 1854–1954*. London: Isis Large Print Books, 2002.

The Durant News. "Durant Boy Member of Hospital Train That Cares For Wounded Soldiers: Capt. John B. Wilkes Transfers Wounded From Battle Action." July 6, 1944.

The Fisherman. "Two UFFO Members Die." February 16, 1945.

Toman, Cynthia. *An Officer and a Lady: Canadian Military Nursing and the Second World War*. Vancouver: UBC Press, 2007.

———. "Front Lines and Frontiers: War as Legitimate Work for Nurses, 1939–1945." *Histoire sociale/Social History*, vol. 40, no. 79 (2007).

Tonopah Daily Bonanza. "Army Hospital Train Carries First Load." January 26, 1917.

Tourret, R. *Allied Military Locomotives of the Second World War: War Department Locomotives* (Abingdon, UK: Tourret Publishing, 1976).

Tremblay, Mary. "The Canadian Revolution in the Management of Spinal Cord Injury." *Canadian Bulletin of Medical History*, vol. 12, no. 1 (Spring 1995): 125–55. https://doi.org/10.3138/cbmh.12.1.125

Tyrer, Nicola. *Sisters in Arms: British Army Nurses Tell Their Story*. London: Weidenfeld & Nicolson Ltd., 2008.

Uek, K. "Former workers, patients remember hospital created for WWII service members." *The Repository*. July 28, 2009. https://www.cantonrep.com/story/news/2009/07/28/former-workers-patients-remember-hospital/47936441007/.

US Army, European Theater of Operations. *That Men Might Live!: The Story of the Medical Service—ETO*. G.I. Stories of the Ground, Air and Service Forces in the European Theater of Operations. Paris: Dupont, 1945. Accessed via the University of Alabama Libraries Special Collections, 1945, Box: 1, Folder: 43., PM-016. http://archives.lib.ua.edu/repositories/3/archival_objects/199263.

US Army. *Bulletin of the United States Army Medical Department*, no. 72 (January 1944).

Vanderklippe, Nathan. "Canada is failing Ukrainians displaced by Russian invasion, former head of Doctors Without Borders says." *Globe and Mail*. April 15, 2022. https://www.theglobeandmail.com/world/article-canada-is-failing-ukrainians-displaced-by-russian-invasion-former-head/.

Walson, Charles M. "Some of the Medical Accomplishments in New York, New Jersey, and Delaware during World War II with Particular Reference to Metropolitan New York." *Military Surgeon*, vol. 100, iss. 4 (April 1947): 294–305. https://doi.org/10.1093/milmed/100.4.294.

Wardlow, Chester. *The Transportation Corps: Movements, Training, and Supply*, vol. 2. Washington, DC: US Army, Office of the Chief of Military History, 1956.

Washington Evening Star. (1941). "Army Hospital Train Will Be Used During Summer Maneuvers." May 19, 1941.

———. "First Overseas-Type Army Hospital Train To Be Exhibited Here." November 22, 1943.

———. "Hundreds Here Visit 10-Car Hospital Train Displayed by Army." November 25, 1943.

Washington Times. "900 Yanks Freed; Arrive in France." December 1, 1918.

West Australian. (1940). Photo caption. June 11, 1940.

Wilmington Morning Star. Photo caption. June 6, 1940.

Winnipeg Free Press. "Wounded Manitoba Soldiers Greeted by Excited Families.", October 21, 1944.

World War II US Medical Research Center. "The Hospital Train in the E.T.O. 1944–1945." https://www.med-dept.com/articles/the-hospital-train-in-the-e-t-o-1944-1945/.

———. "WW2 Military Hospitals: General Introduction." https://www.med-dept.com/articles/ww2-military-hospitals-general-introduction/.

INDEX

1st Battalion of the 16th
  Medical Regiment, 114

Abilene station, 17
ambulance planes, 129
ambulance Trains, 6, 26,
  40–41, 55, 62, 69
American Car & Foundry, 61
American Expeditionary
  Forces (AEF), 6
American Red Cross. *See* Red
  Cross Society
anesthesia, 9, 83, 86
army hospitals, 13
Army Service Forces, 95
Azhnina, Lyudmila (née
  Smirnova), 134

Bayliss, James E., 13
Benet, Laurence V., 30
Benson, Captain, 11
Bessarabia, 40

Big Four, 20
Bluebirds, the, 25, 74, 76
Botterell, E. Harry, 97
British 6th Motor Ambulance
  Convoy, 114
British Ministry of War
  Transport, 68
British Railways. *See under*
  Hospital Trains by Place
British Security Coordination
  (BSC), 115
Bucharest, 40

Camp Hamilton, 24
Camp Lucky Strike, 152
Camp Meade, 22
Canadian Army Medical
  Services, 84
casualties, 33, 42–43, 52, 61,
  66–67, 73, 82, 86, 95, 102,
  103, 111, 113, 115, 117, 123,
  126, 129, 144, 159

Casualty Clearing Station (CCS), 21, 76, 81, 113
chair car. *See* Pullman car
Charing Cross, 19
Chief of Transportation, the, 44
Churchill, A.G. 14
clerks, 159
Colburn, Sam, 22
concentration camps, 2, 6, 10, 70, 132. *See also* Holocaust
conflicts,
    American Civil, the, 21
    Battle of Koeniggraetz, 20
    Crimean War, 19, 24
    D-Day, 42, 67, 109–10, 117
    Dieppe, 18, 67, 69, 103, 116
    Dunkirk, 26
    First World War, 6, 19, 26, 29, 32, 40–44, 55, 60, 62, 69, 100, 142. *See also* World War I
    Franco-Austrian War, 20
    Franco-Prussian War, 22
    Great War, The. *See* First World War
    Operation Little Switch in the Korean War, 151
    Russo–Japanese War, 25
    Second World War, 1, 4–6, 10, 17, 30, 32, 36–37, 41, 44–46, 55, 57, 60, 62, 71, 73, 121, 126, 132, 157, 163, 164. *See also* World War II
Sicilian campaign, 146
Spanish–American War, 22, 39

World War I, 41, 53, 55–57. *See also* First World War
World War II, 53, 78–79, 90, 125, 159. *See also* Second World War
World War Zero. *See* Russo–Japanese War
cooks, 133, 155, 159
Corporal McNally, 66
corpsman, 8
Crissey Field, 7

Darnall, Joseph R., 128
death rates. *See* casualties
Desert Training Center in California, 15
Dillard, James K., 118
diseases, 88
doctors, 1, 25, 40, 48, 72, 83–91
    adapting, 73, 74, 84–85
    Doctors Without Borders, 163
    duties, 51, 83, 86, 90, 91, 129, 163
    interacting with patients, 90, 95, 138
    Navy doctors, 14
    unsung heroes, 84–85, 91, 143, 151, 155, 161
    women doctors, 31.
        See also Gedroits, Vera
Dopke, Gerhard, 160
druggists. *See* pharmacists
Dunbar, Evelyn Mary, 73

Eisenhower, Dwight D., 17

field hospital, 24, 42, 87, 89, 98, 137

Fletcher General Hospital, 95

food rations, 78

Fort Bragg, 13

Fort Douglas, 99

Fort Jackson, 13

Fort McPherson, 13

Foster General Hospital, 118

French railways. *See under* hospital trains by place

FS coaches, 59

gangrene, 88, 89, 127

gas edema serum, 88–89

Gedroits, Vera, 30–31

General John J. Pershing's Mexican Expedition, 39

Geneva Convention, 11, 49

German infantry, 81

German Luftwaffe, 43, 160

Godart, Justin, 30

Grand Junction Railways, the, 19

Halifax, 67, 85, 98, 108

Hamilton, George, 102

Hawk, Alan J., 24

Heaton, Leonard D., 114

Hermann Goring division, the, 160

HMHS *Paris*, 148

Holocaust, 5. *See also* concentration camps

hospital ship, 1, 26–27, 32, 41, 45, 71, 76, 94, 97, 98, 109, 113, 145, 148, 159

hospital train features, 52

commissary department, 28

cost, 32, 49, 135–36,156

design, 11, 20, 28, 32, 34–35, 46, 49, 51–57, 60–61, 63, 66–67, 70, 107, 110

dining car, 10, 15–16, 33, 44, 58, 77, 150, 159

food, 5, 36, 57–59, 147. *See also* food rations

foraging, 78–79

generators, 16, 33

innovation inspired by the war, 37–39, 44, 59, 126

kitchen cars, 10, 13, 15, 16, 29, 33, 44, 45, 48, 54–61, 77, 147, 150

maternity wards, 29, 100

mechanical troubles, 87, 107

mental ward, 57

operating area, 13, 28, 33, 45, 48, 52, 56–58, 60, 81

personnel cars, 11, 48

pharmacy, 15, 16, 52, 57, 59, 159. *See also* pharmacists

quarters, 10, 13, 16, 28, 56, 82, 134, 159

sterilization units, 48, 57, 96

stocking and maintaining, 43

stretchers, 21, 33, 63, 86, 149

technological advancements, 15, 34, 122, 160

types of care, 6, 9, 24, 29, 47,
    38, 91, 126, 129, 131, 147
utility car, 15, 16
ward cars, 15–16, 33, 38, 48,
    52, 59, 77, 149, 159
ward dressing cars, 54, 56,
    58, 59
hospital trains by place,
    Africa, 17, 67, 85, 114, 159,
        162
    Australia, 64–66, 67, 134
    Canada, 63–66, 67, 74, 110,
        149, 152
    China, 162
    Europe, 17, 36, 59, 61, 67,
        69, 71, 77, 85, 98, 100, 108,
        122, 126, 141, 152, 159
    France, 26, 29–30, 70, 109,
        111. *See also* rail toll
    Germany, 122, 125
    India, 9, 162
    Korea, 151
    Malta, 162
    Mexico, 162
    Russia, 31, 162
    Ukraine, 159, 162–63
    United Kingdom, 26,
        67–69, 114, 128
    United States, 12, 29, 32, 45,
        54–59, 61, 63, 67–68,
        75–76, 79, 126, 128
hospital trains,
    as a symbol of hope, 12,
        17–18, 27, 72, 100, 121,
        128, 141–42, 144, 145.

See also effect on morale
    as emblems of peace, 17, 35,
        63, 141
    collecting the fallen, 99,
        102–3
    creation, 19–21, 39, 95
    descriptions, 10, 12–13, 15,
        33–34, 99. *See also* Media
        coverage
    effect on morale, 6, 93,
        95–96, 115, 131, 141
    fading from history, 2, 144,
        151, 155, 157, 162
    freedom or opportunities
        granted women, 3–4,
        30–31, 72–74, 158
    in art, 7, 73, 105
    in literature, 153
    media coverage, 10, 16, 23,
        26, 29, 35, 59, 62, 64, 91,
        95, 112, 130–45, 149, 151.
        See also public view
    neutral ground in war,
        11–12, 29, 32, 105, 106,
        110, 125. *See also* Red
        Cross symbol
    number on board, 11, 22,
        29, 96
    patient accounts, 137, 151
    post-war, 34, 73, 132, 159

    public view, 48, 66, 87, 91,
        99, 122, 130, 136, 144–45,
        149, 157
    relationships, 133, 136, 138, 161

rescuing children, 10
route, 9, 43, 68, 110, 117
use for COVID-19, 159
use in 21st century, 40, 159

immersion foot, 85

Jacksonville, 24

Kelly, Tom, 142

Lady Nelson (Hospital Ship),
110
Laffer, Lorna, 134
Letitia (Hospital Ship), 111
LSTs (Landing Ship, Tank), 127

Mattowitz, Leo, 137
May, Henry C, 118
Medical Department, 15, 27,
31, 41, 46, 53, 57, 122
medical technicians, 159
Medico-Chirurgical hospital, 22
Merritt, C.I., 67
Merritt, F.W.I., 67
mess stewards, 159
Military medical supply
catalogues, 35
Ministry of War, 20, 25, 68
Morgan, J.G., 116, 117

NSW Railways Department,
65
Nazis, 6, 105
Neace, James E., 105

non-medical hospital train
staff, 49, 133. *See also*,
pioneers
nurses, 16, 23, 33, 48, 51-52,
61, 71-82, 148-49, 161, 163
adapting, 1, 73, 74, 85, 86
Canadian military nurses,
76. *See also* Bluebirds,
the
civilian nurses, 45
dangers of the job, 74, 81, 109
defending the trains, 73
duties, 40-45, 51, 72-73, 77,
foraging for food, 78
meals. *See* food rations
military nurses, 13, 14, 45,
109
nurses' quarters, 28, 57
Nursing Sisters. *See*
Bluebirds, the
overwork, 81
post-mortem, 84
post-war difficulties, 132-33
Queen Alexandra's
Imperial Military Nursing
Service, (QAs) 40, 112
uniforms, 48
unsung heroes, 90-91,
143-44, 148, 151, 155
US nurses, 79
Okhrana, 31
orderlies, 13, 35

Panova, Vera, 153-55
paraplegia, 97

Paris, 30, 52, 105, 122, 129

Passenger Branch, 44

penicillin, 127, 137

pharmacists, 135-36, 159. *See also under* Hospital train features

Piecek, Elizabeth "Liz", 79-80

pioneers, 7

porters, 133

prisoners of war, 84, 110, 127, 146

Professor Roux, 31

Pullman Car, 13, 28, 34, 41, 53, 60, 77

Pullman-Standard Car Manufacturing Company, 15, 32, 58, 107

Purser, Thomas, 48

Quebec, 26, 66

Queen Elizabeth (Hospital Ship), 111

Queen Mary (Hospital Ship), 111

Radloff, Ann, 132

rail toll, 69, 112

Railway Executive Committee, 43

Red Cross Society, 7-8, 11, 14, 25, 31, 36, 40, 48, 60, 99, 115, 138

Red Cross symbol, 11, 27, 32, 49, 65, 75, 79, 91, 102, 106, 107, 110, 134. *See also* hospital trains, neutral ground in war

Ringling Brothers Circus, 158

role of women in war, 3, 4, 31, 71-74, 144, 158. *See also* nurses *and* doctors

Rosie the Riveter, 72

Ross, Lady Charles, 26

Ross, Sir Charles, 26

Royal Air Force (RAF), 43, 115

Royal Army Medical Corps (RAMC), 127

Royal Canadian Army Medical Corps, 63-64, 84

sabotage, 106-7

Seaforth Highlanders, 67

Second Kentucky Infantry, 22

Sergeant Ray, 66

shell shock, 101

Shepherd, John, 14

Shirer, William, 115

St. John units, 85

Steuben, 160-61

strafe, 11, 90

stretcher cases, 17, 42, 65, 85, 102, 143, 160. *See also under* Hospital Train Features

stretcher-bearers, 113. *See also under* hospital train features

Surgeon General, 24, 44, 47, 56-57, 114

Surgeon General's Office (SGO), 46, 55-58

Swindon Railway Works, 68

Sylvania Electric Products, Inc., 32

Sylvania installation, 34

theatres of operations. *See* zone of interior

Torkelsen, Helen, 7

trains by name,
   3d Hospital Train, 10
   CPR hospital train, 67. *See also* hospital trains by place
   Canadian National Railways Hospital Car, 149. *See also* hospital trains by place
   Great White Hospital Trains, the, 26
   Hospital Train #23, 105
   Hospital Train Group No. 43, 122
   Hospital Train No. 1, 27
   Kentucky Hospital Train, 22–23
   L-car hospital train, 62
   Ninth Service Command hospital train unit, The, 99
   USA/TC hospital trains, 67

Transportation Corps, 15, 11

train commander, 7–8

UK's Royal Naval Medical Service, 113

United States Army Corps, 32

United States Army Medical Department, 27, 57, 122

United States Army, European Theater of Operations unit, 51, 122

US Navy Hospital, 14

US Surgeon General's Office (SGO). *See* Surgeon General's Office

Ustaše, 6

Victoria Cross, 67

von Mundy, Jaromir Baron, 20

Walker, T.C., 118

walking wounded, the, 12, 42, 52, 83, 96, 101, 102, 143, 151

Walter Reed Army Medical Center, 159

war bonds, 135

War Production Board (WPB), 33–35

ward masters, 159

Washington, 17, 24,

Wicker, Sister G., 81

Wilkes, John B., 15

Williams, U.V., 23

Winter Palace, 31

Wright, Nancy, 142

Yankee Dipper, 60

zone of interior, 10, 47, 68, 75

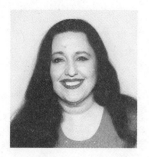

ALEXANDRA KITTY is an award-winning author, educator, and artist whose work has appeared in *Presstime*, *Quill*, *Current*, *Elle Canada*, *Maisonneuve*, *Critical Review*, and *Skeptic*. She was a relationships columnist for the *Hamilton Spectator* and an advice columnist for the Victoria *Times Colonist*. She taught language studies at Mohawk College, writing at the Sheridan Institute, communications at Conestoga College, metalwork arts at Niagara College, and art at the Dundas Valley School of Art. She was the first female recipient of the Arch Award from McMaster University and is the author of a number of books, including *Don't Believe It!: How Lies Become News*; *OutFoxed: Rupert Murdoch's War on Journalism*; *A New Approach to Journalism*; *The Art of Kintsugi*; and *The Dramatic Moment of Fate: The Life of Sherlock Holmes in the Theatre*, among others.